Stop Living Life
Like an Emergency!

Stop Living Life Like an Emergency!

*Rescue Strategies for the Overworked
and Overwhelmed*

Diane Sieg, R.N.

LifeLine
Press

A Regnery Publishing Company
Washington, D.C.

Library of Congress Cataloging-in-Publication Data

Sieg, Diane.

Stop living life like an emergency! : rescue strategies for the overworked and the overwhelmed / Diane Sieg.

p. ; cm.

Includes bibliographical references and index.

ISBN 0-89526-155-3 (alk. paper)

1. Stress management. 2. Type A behavior. [DNLM: 1. Quality of Life--Popular Works. 2. Stress, Psychological--prevention & control--Popular Works. 3. Adaptation, Psychological--Popular Works. 4. Health Behavior--Popular Works. 5. Life Style--Popular Works. WM 172 S5705s 2002] I. Title.

RA785 .S54 2002

613--dc21

2002005789

ISBN: 0-89526-155-3

Published in the United States by
LifeLine Press
A Regnery Publishing Company
One Massachusetts Avenue, N.W.
Washington, DC 20001

Visit us at www.lifelinepress.com

Distributed to the trade by
National Book Network
4720-A Boston Way
Lanham, MD 20706

Book Design and Cover Design by Rich Kershner

Printed on acid-free paper
Manufactured in the United States of America
10 9 8 7 6 5 4 3 2 1

Books are available in quantity for promotional or premium use. Write to Director of Special Sales, Regnery Publishing, Inc., One Massachusetts Avenue, N.W., Washington, D.C. 20001, for information on discounts and terms or call (202) 216-0600.

To Peter,
my best friend, my lover, my life partner

[Contents]

[Acknowledgments]

There are countless people to thank for helping me make this book a reality. Knowing I cannot name every one, I would like to attempt to recognize a few. Thank you Mary LoVerde, my generous mentor and friend, who initiated me into the speaking business and continues to give me something to aspire to. Thank you Shawn Ellis of Premiere Speaker's Bureau, who had enough confidence in me to introduce Karen Anderson to me and start this book in motion. Thank you Karen Anderson, for believing in me and this project as much as I did. Thank you Mike Ward, for giving me this privileged opportunity to work with you and your dynamic staff. Thank you Molly Mullen, my editor, for your patience, enthusiasm, and ongoing encouragement throughout the birth of this book. Thank you LeAnn Thieman, my dear friend and wise mentor, for your ongoing guidance, and unconditional love and support of me and this project from day one. Thank you Molly Hargarten, for your warm support and your frequent endearing comments of "more meat." Thank you Kay Johnson, for your ongoing enlightened perspective and brutal honesty. Thank you Cami Seburn, for your resources and doing the detail work I struggle to do. I have great appreciation for every single red line and comment my aforementioned readers made and however painful they were at the time, your feedback was invaluable to me. Thank you Bev Day, Sue Artt, and Donna Kearns, the three wise women of my Mastermind Group, for supporting me both personally and professionally along this exciting journey. Thank you Jean Bohlke, for generously providing me a safe haven to both begin and complete this book.

I have many mentors and coaches who prodded me along my journey and made it possible for me to share my experiences in this book. Thank you Marsha Earlenbaugh, my career counselor, for giving me the permission I needed to escape the corporate world. Thank you Belle Merwitzer, my life coach, for being the gatekeeper of my dreams and my task-master to help me figure out "my all." Thank you Lou Heckler, my speaking coach, for your creative genius and continued warm and generous support of me. Thank you Joel Roberts, my media coach, for painstakingly browbeating my uniqueness into me. Thank you Marguerite Ham, for keeping me focused and on track with the business of my business. Thank you Pam Gordon, for your wisdom of digging for the word. Thank you Margie Seyfer, for pounding the importance of those critical marketing calls into me. Thank you Diana Scouras, for "getting me" right away and offering me a much-needed new perspective on myself and my life. Thank you Liz De Lange, for introducing me to and supporting me in the powerful practice of yoga. Thank you to my many other mentors, teachers, and friends of Colorado Speakers Association and National Speaker's Association. I would not be where I am today without your generous support and infinite wisdom. Thank you Zach and Matt Sieg, my adored nephews, for reminding me what is really important. Thank you Mom, for your loving support, even if you don't always understand why I do what I do. Many thanks to all of my Lifestyle Counseling clients, who generously shared yourselves with me and demonstrate what is possible when we choose to live differently. Thanks to my fellow health care providers, who worked beside me over the years in hospitals across the country. You have my deepest respect and regard for the significant contributions you make to the noble profession of emergency medicine.

And last but not least, thank you Peter Bohne, my husband, for living this book with me, with your complete confidence and neverending love and support.

[Introduction]

You're running late for work. You forgot to get cupcakes for your son's preschool party and now he's crying hysterically. The dentist appointment you missed three days ago is rescheduled for today, which means you have to cut your conference call short to turn in the proposal by noon. You promised to console a coworker over lunch before her divorce is final and you need to FedEx your Mother's birthday present that you didn't get around to sending last week. You can't find your keys. The cat just threw up—inside your briefcase. You finally get into your car and it won't start. You left your lights on all night and your husband has the jumper cables—in his car parked at the airport.

You are in the throes of emergency living.

Emergency living is life-threatening. It threatens our physical health and emotional well-being, our relationships, and our overall quality of life because it keeps us in a constant state of chaos, crisis, and confusion. We are chronically overworked, overwhelmed, and overdone.

Emergency living leads to emergencies. As an emergency room (ER) nurse for over twenty years, I witnessed overdoses, car accidents, heart attacks, gunshot wounds, severed limbs, and burned bodies. Over the years, I began to realize that, more often than not, the patients I treated created a lot of their own emergencies. Whether it was falling asleep at the wheel because they were exhausted, ignoring warning signs because they were too busy, or rushing to get somewhere because they were running late, their emergency living contributed to the events that brought them to the ER.

Emergency living is treatable. The rescue strategies in this book offer you practical and direct steps and instructions to incorporate into your everyday life—today. Through real life stories, practical prescriptions, and effective exercises, I will show you how to slow down, take time, and take care—all necessary to overcome your life-threatening lifestyle.

In each chapter, I share a life lesson from an ER story that parallels the emergency living in our everyday lives. I give specific action steps you can apply to your own life without having to visit the ER and learn these lessons the hard way. You'll find specific steps on "How do I ...?" in the prescriptions (Rx) section of each chapter.

Every chapter ends with Your Care Plan, a set of exercises for you to put into action what you have learned. You will want to revisit your Care Plan often because your work will change as your life circumstances change. These exercises will enhance your learning experience, improve your success rate of living differently, and help you overcome your life-threatening lifestyle.

I invite you to read this book and begin your path to *Stop Living Life Like an Emergency!*

Chapter 1

Emergency Living

*"Life is what happens to us
while we are making other plans."*
—Thomas La Mance

Why are we all in such a rush? Emergency living is full of chaos, crisis, and panic. It keeps us moving at warp speed, always thinking about the next thing we have to do. We think we have to move faster and faster just to keep up, and we develop a lifestyle to support it.

Our lifestyle is the way we choose to live, the interaction of our thoughts, feelings, attitudes, goals, values, and behaviors. Smoking, being overweight, panic attacks, and codependent relationships are all the symptoms of a much greater problem: emergency living.

When we live life like an emergency, it leads to the destruction and breakdown of every area in our lives, including our physical health, our emotional well-being, and our personal and professional relationships. It may—and often does—even lead to a visit to the emergency room.

ER nurses are known for their autonomy, assertiveness, and technical skills. Their endless courage and compassion for the suffering human spirit are also renown and required, because they are subjected to seeing people in their most vulnerable and dire circumstances. The privilege I had participating in people's lives on such an intimate level provided me with a unique perspective.

I saved many people's lives in the ER, but I didn't feel like I could really change them. My time with them was limited and I usually didn't get an opportunity to follow up with my patients, unless they returned to the ER with another problem. As a Lifestyle Counselor, I could make a bigger and longer-lasting difference in people's lives by counseling them on an ongoing basis. I would much rather work with people before they break down, instead of in a crisis situation in the ER. Today I help my clients change their everyday lives by using the life lessons and survival skills I gleaned from my ER experience.

Living a Life-Threatening Lifestyle

Like so many patients I treated in the ER, my lifestyle counseling clients practice life-threatening lifestyles. The choices they make and the behaviors they follow threaten the quality, and sometimes the quantity, of their lives. Living your life like an emergency is life-threatening.

When you live your life like an emergency:

○ It **threatens your physical health** by depriving you of sleep, leading you down the road to poor nutrition, and making you ignore significant warning signals.

○ It **threatens your emotional well-being** by keeping you distracted, stressed out, and feeling out of control.

  ○ It **threatens your relationships** by preventing you from spending the time and energy that they warrant and deserve.

Staying Busy Being Busy

I was a self-taught expert at "emergency living" long before I ever worked in an emergency room. For almost forty years I stayed busy being busy, overdoing everything from my exercise routines to my social commitments. I was the busiest person I knew, but I still felt like I wasn't doing enough. When we stay busy being busy we don't have time—for anything. Not even to take care of ourselves in a real emergency!

A fifty-year-old man dressed in an expensive three-piece suit rushed through the ER doors with a tall, attractive blonde woman on his arm. While checking his cell phone for messages, he simultaneously spoke to me in a swift and sharp voice: "I'm here only because my wife insisted on it. I'm having a little indigestion this morning, but I really don't have time for this. I have a plane to catch in less than two hours."

His skin color was gray and I noticed beads of sweat dripping down his forehead. My further questioning revealed he had been up most of the night with chest heaviness and shortness of breath. He had chewed several antacid tablets at home with no effect and now felt nauseated.

He admitted to being under a lot of stress recently with his promotion to National Sales Manager and had started smoking again. All of his symptoms were classic warning signs of a heart attack, including his denial that anything was wrong with him.

He was fortunate that his wife insisted he come in, even though he didn't have time for it. He required open-heart surgery and was operated on the next day.

This patient knew he was stressed, smoked too much, and wasn't taking care of himself. He had plenty of other warning signs for his heart attack that he also chose to ignore: the "heart-burn" that didn't go away even after taking antacids, the profuse sweating, nausea, and shortness of breath—all classic signs of a pending heart attack. The most obvious warning sign he had was his denial that anything was wrong. He didn't really "have time for this" since he was on his way to a business meeting.

His emergency living affected him physically by landing him in the ER with a heart attack. It affected him emotionally by causing him a lot of stress, which contributed to his heavy smoking. His life-threatening lifestyle had a significant effect on his family relationships, because he traveled frequently and often missed his kids' soccer games and school plays. He didn't really have time for a heart attack, but had he not come in to the hospital, he would have died on the way to his business meeting.

Just like the warning signs of a heart attack, there are classic warning signs of emergency living that show up when we're trying to do too much, too fast, too often. Like the warning signs of a heart attack, we may deny our emergency living, until something serious happens to force us to pay attention.

The Seven Warning Signs of Emergency Living

1 You are always running late—just a little.

2 You have accumulated piles everywhere: piles of clothing, piles of paper, and piles of piles you are going to get to someday.

3 You find yourself in one of three modes: "hurry up," "catch up," or "fed up."

4 You constantly lose things: your glasses, your car keys, even your mind. Losing your mind includes forgetting your best friend's birthday, avoiding your neighbor in the grocery store because you can't remember his name, or putting out your trash on the wrong day.

5 You have no patience for heavy traffic, grocery lines, and anything else that "takes too long."

6 You pride yourself on not only how much you get done, but how fast you do it.

7 You frequently find yourself saying, "When things *slow down*, I'm really going to…

      Exercise…

        Get more rest…

          Take better care of myself…"

How many of these signs do you recognize in yourself? If you find yourself experiencing *even one* of these warning signs, you are at high risk for emergency living. If you're familiar with two or more, you are already living your life like an emergency!

Emergency Living Personalities

We all have certain innate personality traits that can predispose us to emergency living. These traits can dictate many of the decisions we make in both our personal and our professional lives. Far from being a negative, most of these characteristics are very admirable, and the people who have them are high-energy and driven in whatever they do. It's when they're taken to the extreme that they lead to emergency living.

The Controller

We all need to feel like we are in control to some extent—that's normal and healthy. But we get into trouble when we feel like we are the only ones who can do it "right." When you think you are the only one who can do the laundry, set the table, and run the meeting most efficiently, you will most likely end up doing it all, or at least trying to do it all.

The Perfectionist

When you can't say something is "good enough" the way it is, until you have struggled with it, done it over several times, or given it 150 percent, you are obsessed with doing a perfect job. Being obsessive about perfection requires more time and energy than you probably allow, which puts you at a faster pace just to keep up.

The Driver

These individuals are highly motivated by their own egos and value themselves for what they do and how much they get done.

They are more critical of themselves than anyone else would ever be. They often have unrealistic expectations. They tend to set high standards not only for themselves, but for everyone around them.

The Action Person

While many of us are more comfortable to stand back and watch something, these individuals are the ones who will jump in. They prefer to *do* rather than to *be*. Obviously, these traits are critical to ER personnel, but some situations in our everyday lives warrant taking a step back and evaluating the situation without doing something immediately. Sometimes we need to just stand there.

The Adrenaline Junkie

These individuals tend to thrive on lots of activity and the panic, chaos, and crisis management that go along with it. They create their own stressful situations by the choices they continue to make to meet their need for excitement. These situations, which can feel like "emergencies," are characterized by unhealthy relationships, ridiculous schedules, and impractical commitments.

The Risk Taker

Just like the individuals who thrive on adrenaline and excitement, risk taking can provide the same kind of stimulation. These individuals think nothing of taking huge risks in their lives physically, socially, or financially. The risk taking gives them an edge, and they feel the boredom of living in a safe, predictable, and stable world would be much more stressful.

The Impatient

These individuals want it *now*. They live in the moment and want results in the moment. They can be impatient and even impulsive about spending their money, getting involved in relationships, and making other significant decisions. They are not long-term thinkers and are more inclined to think about next week's vacation than about retirement.

The Rescuer

The rescuer is the person who is first to volunteer to work late, bake the cookies, walk the neighbor's dog, or do anything else to save the day. They frequently attract very needy people and usually have several projects or people they are trying to help. And since they find it very difficult to say no to a commitment or request, they are the first ones asked.

The Difference Maker

When you need to be needed, you will always find who and what needs you. You will volunteer, work, and socialize at levels you know are making a difference, in your career, your personal life, or in the world—be it politics, religion, or community action. You are committed to helping others no matter what it takes, and sometimes at all costs.

People with these personality traits can be very successful because they create positive outcomes when their energy is channeled appropriately. But when they cross the line and go to the extreme with these traits, emergency living begins.

Emergency living sneaks up on us and becomes a pattern, a habit, and a familiar way of life. We often don't realize how frantically we are living until something serious happens to get our attention. Until we are forced to stop by an illness, an injury, or another life-changing event, we just keep on going.

Break Through Before You Break Down

The whole premise of *Stop Living Life Like an Emergency!* is to do it before you end up in the emergency room. You don't have to wait for an illness, an injury, or anything else to break you down before you break through. You can change the way you live today, or you can continue to have emergencies in your life.

I am very familiar with the personality traits that predispose me to emergency living. I humbly share many similarities with the perfectionist, the driver, the controller, and the adrenaline junkie. Working in the ER held a lot of interest for me because of the intense element of surprise, the unpredictable environment, and the frequent adrenaline surges. With my hard-driving ambition, I have a tendency to overdo things in my life, like my work, my social commitments—even my exercise.

My compulsive exercising caused me frequent injuries to my back, knees, and ankles, and I became quite well known to the physical therapy department at my local hospital. Unfortunately, it took an incapacitating event for me to realize there was a correlation between my chronic injuries and the way I was living. I had to *break down* before I could *break through*.

I started out with a sore foot in the spring and ended up with a full leg cast for the entire summer. This was totally preventable had I just given in to my injury and followed the doctor's orders to "take it easy."

When I gave up my formal exercising I really thought I was "taking it easy." Even though I stopped kickboxing and running, I continued to drive, work my twelve-hour shifts in the ER, and carry on my everyday activities.

The final straw was when I refused a wheelchair at the Denver airport, one of the biggest airports, with the longest concourses, in the world. That final shenanigan left me with both feet hurting and one leg in a cast, forcing me to stop and surrender to my circumstances. I gave up all driving, working, and walking anywhere, except for around the house. I was even reduced to letting my seventy-year-old mother push me through the mall in a wheelchair.

This injury to my feet was the most incapacitating of all of my injuries. It was a frustrating, devastating, agonizing… gift. I found myself with a lot of time on my hands and this gift of time allowed me to stop and really examine my life. What was all of my running around about? Where was I going? What was I doing?

Brake Before You Break

My agonizing gift required me to let go of my familiar theme of "*more, better, faster.*" I learned patience because everything took me so much longer to do. I learned surrender because I was finally forced to face my circumstances. I learned how to take care of myself because I wanted to heal. I learned all of this because I was forced to *slow down* in my life.

You don't have to wait for a serious illness, injury, or life-changing event before you decide to *slow down* in your life. If you heed your own warning signs of emergency living, you can *break through* before you *break down*.

How can I slow down in my life?
———————— [Rx] ————————

- Recognize that slowing down can be initially uncomfortable.
- Speak slower and softer.
- Eat and drink slower.
- Drive slower.
- Take a pause between phrases, tasks, and stressful moments.
- Stop for five minutes in your day to be quiet and still.
- Listen more intently to others with a quiet and open mind.
- Do one thing at a time and really focus on that one thing.
- Take a real "breather" by inhaling a full, deep belly-breath and exhaling long and slow.
- Observe the haste of the people and activity around you and notice how you feel about their frenzy.

[Your Care Plan]

1 List your warning signs for emergency living:

2 List your personality traits that predispose you to emergency living:

3 We all have our own belief systems about slowing down in our lives. What are you fears or concerns about slowing down? *Example: I'm afraid if I slow down I won't get it all done.*

My biggest fear about slowing down is:

What could you lose by slowing down?

What could you gain by slowing down?

_____

_____

_____

4 Look at the list of slowing-down activities. Do you have any
   other ideas to help you slow down? Choose one activity or
   idea to practice for a whole day, just as an experiment. At the
   end of that day, take stock of how you feel after slowing down
   this part of your life.

   Did you have any discomfort or anxiety?

   Did you notice anything you haven't noticed before?
   What was it?

   Was your day any different?

   Were you any different?

5 For the next ten days, pick one slowing-down activity to
   focus on each day, just as an experiment. Write yourself a
   note to help remind you which activity to practice that day
   and put it somewhere you can see it all day long. Notice
   which activity is the most difficult and which one is the eas-
   iest for you. After your ten-day experiment, identify which
   one(s) you can incorporate into your everyday life.

Chapter 2

Triage

"It is not enough that you are busy.
The question is, what are you so busy about?"
—Henry David Thoreau

When someone comes to the ER as a patient, the first person they speak to is the triage nurse, who listens to what the patient says, and also to what they don't say. The triage nurse is highly skilled at assessing the situation of the patient very quickly and after listening carefully to their story, she determines if immediate attention is needed, or if they can wait and be taken care of later. Sometimes, much later.

Just like triaging patients in the ER, we have to sort through our own lives by itemizing, prioritizing, and scrutinizing our everyday activities. We may talk about how important our health, our family, or our faith is to us, but how much time do we *really* spend on them? When we don't sort our lives, we end up spending a lot of time and energy on things that just aren't that important. The ER could never function effectively without triaging patients according to their level of urgency.

A woman in her seventies gingerly walked into the triage area complaining of a "tight chest." Short of breath from just talking, she reported taking three nitroglycerin tablets under her tongue at home without any effect. With her previous cardiac history and her current symptoms, I took her back to a treatment room immediately, even though she said, "I can wait if you need me to."

The next patient I triaged was a small man, fully outfitted in fishing gear, with a fishhook lodged in his index finger. He was adamant about immediately letting me know he was a "physician from a large medical center back East." I asked him to have a seat and wait.

After he got up several times to ask me how much longer it would be, I gently reminded him how fortunate he was to be waiting, instead of being treated for a heart attack. He sheepishly sat back down.

This is triage at work in the ER.

What happens when we don't sort our fishhooks from our heart attacks, when we don't take the time to sort through our daily activities and prioritize our commitments? We get distracted, we have no sense of what is most important, we find ourselves unrealistically overcommitted. No wonder we're so tired!

There are many reasons why we get worn out and worn down, and lose our perspective and our ability to make the best choices when we don't sort through our lives.

Everything Takes Longer

Getting our kids ready for school, driving across town, or stopping at the grocery store all take longer than the time we usually allot. Actually, most things take nearly twice as long as what we plan on. This is why so many of us are chronically running late.

To stop running late we have to be realistic about how long things take. We not only have to allow time for the actual activity, we have to allow transition time from one activity to the next, and account for all of life's unforeseen circumstances such as a ten-car pileup on the freeway, treacherous weather, and other people's emergencies.

If you are someone who is always late you must acknowledge that when you are late for anything, you send the message that your time is more valuable than the person forced to wait for you. I had a client who was chronically late because if you asked her how long it took to get anywhere in town, she thought it was five minutes. Even if it took nine, or fifteen, or twenty-two, she still allowed only five minutes.

People who are chronically late will always make one more stop they think they have time for when they aren't running late, which, of course, makes them late after all. Being early shows a real respect for the other person and gives you time to take a breath and relax for a few moments before your meeting or appointment.

Procrastination Leads to Complication

Procrastination is the root of many evils. Whether it is holiday shopping, paying the electric bill, or planning for a trip, procrastination always catches up to you. Procrastination complicates our lives because it reduces us to doing a search-and-rescue mission for that one-of-a-kind gift, deliver bills in person,

or cram in last-minute panic packing. The longer we procrastinate, the farther behind we get, the more overwhelmed we get,
the more immobilized we get...and the farther behind we get.

There is a reason we procrastinate, and even though we may
not be conscious of it, it is serving us in some way. We may really detest holiday shopping, so we wait until the last minute
when we have few choices available and we're short on time. We
may be resentful of paying the electric company one-third of our
salary, so we get a sense of vindication in holding out on them.
We may be uncertain of what we want to pack so we put off
making any decisions about what to take on that business trip.
If you can determine why you are procrastinating by figuring out
how it is serving you, you'll be more successful in avoiding it.

Interruptions Are Expensive

If we looked closely at how we spend our time and energy, we
would see that more of our time is spent trying to get around to
doing something than actually *doing* it. The constant interruptions in our daily lives—phone calls, pages, e-mails, voice mails,
faxes—often intrude on our more important activities, and we
don't usually account for how costly they are to our schedule.
Interruptions take away our time, our energy, and, most importantly, our flow. These new demands have to be managed too,
and then it takes us more time to get back to trying to do what
we were doing in the first place.

We allow ourselves to be interrupted. We are not treating
whatever we are trying to do with very much importance when
we allow interruptions. It is easy to forget we are the ones to de-

cide how and when we want to respond. This includes returning e-mail, phone calls, and any other correspondence.

There is, of course, business etiquette for returning correspondence, but there is also a large cost to our business, family, and sanity, for being continuously interrupted. When I was writing this book, I turned off the ringer on my phone every morning between 8 A.M. and 12 noon, letting the answering machine pick up my messages, because even a short phone conversation was a distracting interruption to my creative flow. I returned phone calls in the afternoon and most of my friends and associates caught on quickly and waited to call me then.

Overscheduling Is Overwhelming

Some of us think we always "should" be able to do more, so we consistently overschedule ourselves. Then we wind up feeling discouraged and defeated when we can't get it all done. We have to accept the reality of our time and energy limitations and schedule ourselves accordingly.

Take a look at your own schedule for next week: How does it feel? Is it overwhelming or is it exciting to you? Are you looking forward to the coming week or just hoping to get through it?

We all know people who overschedule themselves. Many times they are the same ones who are chronically late, are big-time procrastinators, and always allow themselves to be interrupted. We can get so used to being overwhelmed with our schedule, we forget we have choices. We may not even know how to do it differently.

We need to be honest with ourselves about our reserves of time and energy. We have to learn to limit our social engagements, evening activities, and other commitments that put our schedule at risk for being overwhelmed. When we take the time to sort our life and determine what activities are most important to us, we can stop overscheduling and we can stop feeling so overwhelmed.

The Triage Tag

Sorting is not just about getting organized. It is determining what is most important and then eliminating, terminating, or delegating the rest of the less important activities. We have to determine what really needs our immediate attention and what is most important, and what can wait, or be discarded altogether. While it may be easier to sort our fishhooks from our heart attacks, it is more challenging to figure out how to sort our day-to-day activities.

Triage tags are used by the ER for disasters, accidents, or any situation that could result in a potentially high number of casualties. The triage tag is a physical tag attached to each patient with the identifying information. We sort each patient by a priority ranging from one to four, according to the status of their injuries and their treatment needs. The triage tag ensures each patient is treated in the most appropriate and efficient way possible.

When a school bus carrying fifty-two Girl Scouts rolled over into the river, we used the triage tag system to sort each girl by priority for treatment. Even though the girls were primarily cold and scared, the triage tags proved very useful. Each girl was quickly assessed and had the appropriate tag attached to her. The categories we used were as follows:

- o **Immediate** is a Priority One. This is an unstable or potentially unstable patient whose condition will deteriorate without immediate attention. The girl with abdominal pain and a low blood pressure was a Priority One and was treated first.

- o **Delayed** is a Priority Two. This is a stable patient whose treatment may be delayed. The girl with a swollen ankle was Priority Two and was treated second.

- o **Minor** is a Priority Three. This is a stable patient who may or may not need treatment. The girl with superficial scratches on her leg was a Priority Three and was treated third.

- o **Deceased** is a Priority Four. Fortunately, we didn't have anyone to assign this category, but if we did, she would have been a Priority Four and handled last for obvious reasons.

We can use the Triage Tag system with our daily activities by sorting them according to their level of importance in our lives:

- o **Immediate:** These activities are Priority One and are the *most important* in our lives. If these activities do not get immediate attention, our life situation deteriorates. Eating meals is categorized as a Priority One.

○ **Delayed:** These activities are Priority Two and are *important*, but not *most important*. They need to be handled, but can be delayed or done at a different time. Grocery shopping can be scheduled at a different time.

○ **Minor:** These activities are Priority Three and are *less important*. Someone else can handle these activities, or they need to be discarded altogether. Some of the endless errands we seem to have on our list, like picking up dry cleaning, could be discarded by using a delivery service.

○ **Deceased:** These activities are Priority Four and are *not important* at all. These activities need to be discarded. These are the activities that are draining you of your time, and are things like looking for a lost sock, or going back home for something you forgot.

Eliminate, Delegate, or Terminate

Once we sort our life activities using the Triage Tag system, we can choose to spend our time and energy on the (1) *most important* and (2) *more important* ones. This requires us to give up and get rid of the (3) *less important* or (4) *not important* activities.

For most of us, giving anything up is difficult. We like to believe we are capable of doing it all. What really ends up happening is we *try* to do it all, and get ourselves exhausted and frustrated in the process. We can give up and get rid of our (3) and (4) activities three ways:

○ **Elimination (E):** Removing the activity from our schedule immediately.

○ Delegation (D): Assigning the activity or transferring the responsibility to someone else.

○ Termination (T): Scheduling or ending the activity on a specified date and time.

As a Lifestyle Counselor, I help people manage themselves and their lives better, which almost always involves sorting. Leslie initially came to see me for weight management, but after our first visit it was clear her extra weight was only a symptom of her real issues.

Leslie and her husband were both full-time physicians and had two small children. Between taking calls, scheduling child care, and the normal stresses of being an oncologist, Leslie was totally overwhelmed by her life. Exhausted and frustrated, she felt herself slipping away as her life continued to spin out of control. Leslie needed to sort through her life and actively choose how she spent her time and energy.

The Activity Log

Leslie's first assignment for sorting her life was to keep a log of her daily activities. I asked her to write down everything she did in thirty-minute intervals from the moment she got up until she went to bed. I encouraged her to keep the log handy and make entries in it throughout the day for the most accurate tracking.

The best way to examine any behavior, such as your eating habits, mood swings, or how you spend your time, is to write it down. This lets you look at the reality of what you do, how often you do it, and how long it takes you. As painful as it can be to write things down, it is very revealing. After Leslie kept a log for a week, I showed her how to sort her activities using the Triage Tag system.

Below is an example of Leslie's log and how she sorted her activities. Her (3) and (4) activities are in boldface for easier reference.

Activity Log

Activity	Importance (1-4)	Eliminate Delegate Terminate
0530 Alarm, shower, started coffee	2	
0600 Picked out clothes for day (kids & me)	2	
0630 Woke up kids, got kids dressed, **looked for lost shoe**	3	T
0700 Breakfast, fed dog, packed lunches, **looked for keys**	3	E
0730 Drove kids to school, got gas, **back home for "show and tell project"**	4	E
0830 Arrived at office **20 minutes late**	4	T
1730 Left office late, pick up dry cleaning, **FedEx late birthday present**	3	D
1800 Grocery store	2	
1830 **Threw dinner together,** everyone hungry and tired	4	D

Refer to Leslie's activity log to see how she got rid of her (3) and (4) activities. She specifically eliminated, delegated, or terminated the *less important* and *not important* activities by:

- Getting rid of the clutter around her house by scheduling a pick-up date for the Salvation Army. (*Elimination*)

- Laying out everyone's clothes, shoes, and socks—including her own, the night before. (*Termination*)

- Having meals prepared by someone else or ordering out on long work days. (*Delegation*)

- Scheduling errands logistically and sticking to only those scheduled errands. (*Termination*)

- Utilizing delivery services to minimize errands.(*Delegation*)

[Your Care Plan]

1 For seven days, log your own activity in thirty-minute intervals using the blank log provided. Try not to change your activity, just witness it and record it. This will reveal how you are *really* spending your time and energy.

2 Sort each of the activities from your log according to their importance: (1) *most important,* (2) *more important,* (3) *less important,* and (4) *not important.* Remember that everything you do cannot be *most important.* If fifty-two Girl Scouts from a rollover bus can be sorted, so can your daily activities.

3 Look at the activities you labeled as (3) and (4). Decide how you will get rid of them in your life by elimination (E), delegation (D), or termination (T). You don't have to get rid of them all at once, but at least identify your plan.

4 After you eliminate at least one *less important* and one *not important* activity, re-evaluate your schedule. How does it feel? You can log and sort your activities whenever your life is feeling overwhelming or out of control. You can also use this form to examine specific behaviors such as what you eat, when you exercise, or how much money you spend.

Activity Log

Activity	Importance (1-4)	Eliminate Delegate Terminate
0530		
0600		
0630		
0700		
0730		
0800		
0830		
0900		
0930		
1000		

1030 _____

1100 _____

1130 _____

1200 _____

1230 _____

1300 _____

1330 _____

1400 _____

1430 _____

1500 _____

1530 _____

1600 _____

1630 _____

1700 _____

1730 _____

1800 _____

1830 _____

1900 _____

1930 _____

2000 _____

2030 _____

Activity Log (continued)

Activity	Importance (1-4)	Eliminate Delegate Terminate
2100		
2130		
2200		
2230		
2300		
2330		
2400		

Chapter 3

Assessment

"Who looks outside dreams;
Who looks inside wakes."
—C.G. Jung

When a patient comes into the ER, whether they've been involved in a rollover car accident or have a sore throat, the first thing the nurse does is assess the patient's status. The assessment includes a medical history and a physical examination. If they are able to respond, the patient is asked about their chief medical complaint and what brought them to the ER, any medications they may be taking, and what allergies they have.

The physical exam consists of taking the patient's vital signs, starting with blood pressure, heart rate, temperature, respiration rate, and sometimes oxygen saturation levels to assess their breathing status. The physical exam also involves evaluation of the area associated with the patient's chief complaint. If the patient comes in having difficulty breathing, we listen to their heart and lungs; if they have a crushed leg, we check their pulses and levels of sensation.

Many emergency rooms use SOAP notes, a documentation system for assessing the patient. SOAP refers to the **Subjective**, what the patient is saying; the **Objective**, what the health care provider sees or notices on evaluation; the **Assessment**, the main problem(s) identified; and the **Plan**, the intended treatment. A SOAP note for an ER patient might look like this:

- o **Subjective.** What the patient says:
  "My jaw is killing me"

- o **Objective.** What the health care provider sees on evaluation:
  Forty-six-year-old obese man with jaw pain and significant cardiac history

- o **Assessment.** The main problem(s) identified:
  Alteration in comfort due to possible heart attack

- o **Plan.** The intended treatment:
  Admit to hospital to rule out heart attack

Making a comprehensive assessment requires good listening, interviewing, and physical exam skills and concentrated focus on the patient. The assessment is fundamental in patient care because it provides critical information to allow the medical staff to choose the right diagnostic tests, medications, and treatments needed. In the midst of an often chaotic scene—crash carts racing, sirens blaring, and people screaming at any given time—the ER nurse has to stop and take the time and attention required to focus on the patient assessment.

If we live life like an emergency, we need to do an assessment of our own everyday lives in order to wake up, pay attention, and take a good honest look at ourselves. Just like in the

ER, an accurate self-assessment requires us to stop and focus on our own lives.

We can stop in our everyday lives by being still, being quiet, and just *being*. Stopping allows us to check in with ourselves. Stopping grounds us, centers us, rescues us from all the stimulation from the outside world, and allows us to retreat to the inside.

When we don't take the time to stop in our lives, we don't pay attention; we move faster and faster to keep up. We just keep on going even if it's unhealthy, destructive, or lethal. The story below is an extreme case of what happened to someone who did not stop and assess himself, even in the face of life-threatening circumstances. He brings a whole new meaning to sleepwalking through life and being in denial.

A forty-six-year-old man drove himself to the ER at 2:00 a.m. complaining of jaw pain. He said, "I just need a couple of pain pills so I can get some sleep."

His weight was 376. His blood sugar was 326; the normal range is 60–100. He was a diabetic and admitted to "having a few chocolate bunnies on the way to the hospital." His oxygen level was 71 percent; normal is 90 percent or higher. "I'm having a really hard time quitting smoking," he said.

He couldn't remember when his last two heart attacks were, but he did recall having bypass surgery on his forty-second birthday. With an abnormal electrocardiogram reading, his low oxygen level, and his medical history, he didn't go anywhere that night. He was admitted to the hospital for a possible heart attack.

The next day his lab results confirmed a heart attack and he was scheduled for a cardiac catheterization to study the arteries in his heart. But it was April 15—tax day. Despite being told he'd just had a heart attack, he signed himself out of the hospital against all medical advice and went home to do his taxes.

I realize this is a ridiculously extreme example of someone not paying attention to virtually every area of his life. He has obviously not taken the time to stop and assess himself even in the face of all his serious health issues. But a lot of us have areas in our lives we don't pay enough attention to. What will it take for *you* to stop?

The Power of Stopping

Stopping is an opportunity to center and focus on ourselves, a form of meditation in which we allow our minds to be quiet and still. John Kabat Zinn says, "meditation is paying attention on purpose, in the present moment, non-judgmentally." We stop by focusing on our breath to quiet our busy minds and rest, not only physically, but emotionally. Stopping gives us the opportunity to listen. I'm not talking about all the mindless chatter and the endless "to do" lists that run through our heads all day. I'm talking about listening to our hearts, our inner voice, our intuition. We develop our intuition by taking the time to listen to it and learning to trust it.

We have all been in situations when we didn't listen to our inner voice. Afterward, we berated ourselves, saying "I just had a feeling that…" or "I knew I should have…." When we use our intuition, we stay congruent with what we know and what we do. Intuition is just as invaluable in our everyday lives as it is in the ER.

The patient was thirty-eight years old and had no risk factors for heart disease. He appeared exceptionally healthy as he casually walked in complaining of vague abdominal and back pain. His blood pressure was a little high, but his color was good, and he wasn't in any obvious distress.

The nurse who checked him in had strong assessment skills and a feeling—that gut feeling we don't always want to listen to—that this man was not going to do well. She called the Intensive Care Unit for backup and paged the cardiac surgeon. In less than fifteen minutes, the man's pain increased significantly, his blood pressure dropped to almost nothing, and he lost consciousness.

Fortunately, he was taken to surgery immediately for repair of a ruptured aortic aneurysm. This is a weak spot in the wall of the heart that can burst, depleting the blood supply to the rest of the body. Aortic aneurysms have a very high mortality rate, but by doing a thorough assessment and listening to her intuition, that ER nurse saved this young man's life.

We can stop anywhere—in our office, in our home, or outdoors in nature. The only requirement for this quiet and uninterrupted time is our willingness to do it. Stopping for as little as five minutes a day can give us incredible self-awareness by allowing us to be quiet and escape the constant stimulation of the outside world. It also calms us from the inside out because we often carry the noise and distractions within us.

> I was speaking to a group of top sales performers in a pharmaceutical company when one of the sales representatives shared with us how stopping helped him through graduate school. He has severe attention-deficit disorder, a condition that makes it very hard to focus and concentrate on one thing for an extended period of time. He learned the power of stopping from of one of his professors.
>
> Every evening, before he started studying, he stopped for twenty minutes to quiet and calm his mind. He said he still practices this exercise because it makes such a difference in his ability focus on his work. It apparently continues to benefit him, as shown by his outstanding sales performance.

If stopping is powerful enough to help someone with severe attention-deficit disorder get through graduate school, then imagine how powerful it can be for you.

Permission to Stop

Stopping is not an easy thing for us to do because it isn't encouraged or supported in our society today. Who has the time to stop these days with so much to do?

But I don't think we have time *not* to stop. *We need to stop to keep us going.*

When I present my program, I lead my audience in a stopping exercise. I play a CD of soft flute music, and ask them to close their eyes and spend a few minutes checking in with themselves. There are always a few who are visibly uncomfortable, squirming in their chairs and sneaking a peak just to make sure everyone else is doing it. One woman told me it was the longest five minutes of her life!

I have to admit I was pretty nervous when I first started asking big kahuna investment bankers or large, burly construction workers to stop. My concerns were totally unwarranted because not only did they really get into it, they thanked me after my program for giving them the opportunity.

Like any new behavior, stopping requires practice. And to practice stopping requires us to give ourselves permission. Author David Kundtz gives us that permission beautifully in his book, *Everyday Serenity.*

Permission to Stop

"Unnecessary self-restrictions and false guilt burden many of us and keep us from the peaceful times we yearn for. Quiet time to be alone is not an optional nicety; nor is it just for the retired, the lazy, or those naturally inclined. It is for all of us. It is valuable time well spent. And above all, it needs no justification other than its own noble purpose: to become more fully awake and to remember what you most need to remember about yourself and your life."

[Your Care Plan]

The first step to self-assessment is learning how to stop. Don't worry about doing it right; there is no right or wrong way to do it. Know that it may be uncomfortable initially and that some days will be easier than others. Of all of the exercises in this book, I feel the strongest about this one. I give you not only the permission, but my absolute encouragement and support to do this exercise and stop, just as an experiment.

1 Pick a time in the day when you can stop for five minutes, preferably the same time every day, for the next seven days. I suggest early mornings for two reasons: There is less opportunity for interruption and distraction, and it will set the tone for the rest of your day if you practice stopping first thing in the morning.

   Find a quiet and comfortable place for yourself. You may even want to designate a special area in your home for stopping. If you decide to use music, play something without lyrics or a familiar melody. Set a timer for five minutes (or however long you decide) so you won't get distracted checking your watch.

   Sit in a restful position in a chair or on the floor. Close your eyes and start to focus on your breathing. Notice your inhalation, the breath coming in, as well as your exhalation, the breath going out. To help you focus on your breathing, count your inhalations up to ten, and then count back down to one as you exhale. If your busy mind starts sneaking in, making lists and reminding you of all the other things you should be doing, gently push it aside and return the focus to your breathing.

For the next seven days examine and document how stopping feels for you both before and after the exercise and note the level of difficulty you have with the practice. Level 1 is very easy, level 3 is neutral, level 5 is very hard.

Example:

	Feelings Before	Level of Difficulty Stopping (1–5)	Feelings Afterward
Day 1	Unsettled	5–Very hard	More calm

	Feelings Before	Level of Difficulty Stopping (1–5)	Feelings Afterward
Day 1			
Day 2			
Day 3			
Day 4			
Day 5			
Day 6			
Day 7			

2 The second step for self-assessment is to use the SOAP charting system for yourself after you complete the stopping exercise.

The (S) **Subjective** is pretty straightforward. It is what we think and say to ourselves during our stopping. It is a

subjective opinion or statement we make about ourselves and it usually is vague and broad, but the more specific, the better.
Example:
Broad: *"I just don't feel good"*
Better: *"I am really tired."*

The (O) **Objective** is a little less obvious. It is hard to be objective with ourselves. We may think we know why we are feeling a certain way, but it usually takes more investigation. As the story on page 31 illustrates, it is easy for us to deny what is really going on in our lives without a thorough self-assessment. It is helpful to keep asking ourselves deeper questions.
Example:
Why am I so tired?
"Because I'm not getting enough sleep."

Why aren't I getting enough sleep?
Because I get home from work late all wound up and unable to go to bed for hours. After watching TV and eating too much, I go to bed and toss and turn all night. I wake up several times because I am so stressed out about my personality conflicts with my boss. I am tired because my high stress level is not allowing me to have restful sleep, and also because I am so stressed during the day that I am always on edge.

The (A) **Assessment** is an overall evaluation based on your subjective and objective statements.
Example: My lack of confrontational skills is interfering with my quality of life. I cannot sleep because I feel so stressed.

The (P) **Plan** is what you can do to treat this problem.
Example: I will set up a meeting with my boss to discuss some specific issues I am concerned with—for example, I need more resources, my deadline needs to be pushed back, or I need to find another job.

Write your own **SOAP** note right after you practice your stopping exercise.

(S) **Subjective:** What were you thinking or saying to yourself?

_____

_____

(O) **Objective:** What is going on in your life that contributes to your thinking this way?

_____

_____

(A) **Assessment:** Write your own assessment or conclusion based on your subjective and objective statements:

_____

_____

(P) **Plan:** Identify an action plan to treat this issue:

_____

_____

3 The third step for self-assessment is evaluation. After your seven days of practice ask yourself these questions:

Is your stopping working? Is it effective?

Is it any easier?

What makes it easier or more difficult?

Are your days any different?

Do you feel any different about the exercise?

What have you learned about yourself?

Have you been surprised by anything that came up for you?

As you continue to practice stopping, you can always work up to longer than five minutes. You will find the more you practice, the more comfortable you become with it, but there will still be days when it is more difficult than others. Increasing your stopping time is not required because even five minutes a day will give you incredible focus and clarity by allowing you to be quiet and listen.

Chapter 4

Hyperventilation

"Fear is excitement without the breath."

–Fritz Perls, M.D.

*T*o *take in our breath more fully* is to literally take in our life more fully. Even though breathing is vital to our existence, most of us take it for granted and utilize only one-sixth of our total lung capacity. Many of us are unaware of all the repercussions of not breathing to our full capacity. When we breathe shallow and fast (hyperventilate) or hold our breath we compromise our breathing, and we compromise our lives.

Hyperventilation is a common occurrence in the ER. It can be caused by many circumstances including fever, asthma, and a head injury, but the most common cause is acute anxiety and pain. When we are stressed or in pain, we respond by tightening and constricting our entire bodies, which hinders our ability to take in full, deep breaths. We compensate by hyperventilating, thus setting up a vicious cycle, because our anxiety and pain actually increase the faster we breathe.

The ER patient who is hyperventilating first needs to become aware of her breathing and then be coached into breathing deeper and slower. Deep breathing alleviates some of the stress

and pain before other treatments such as medications or procedures can be effective.

> A wrangler dressed in full gear with chaps and boots wheeled
> his twenty-year-old girlfriend into the ER. Doubled over in a
> wheelchair, she moaned with severe abdominal pain. They
> both worked at a ranch outside of town and a horse had
> kicked her in the stomach moments ago.
>
> She was breathing fast and shallow and shivered uncon-
> trollably, complaining of dizziness and tingling around her
> mouth and fingers. These secondary symptoms were caused
> by hyperventilation due to her pain and anxiety.
>
> The first priority was to get her to slow down and deepen
> her breathing to help her relax. I encouraged her to take in full,
> deep belly-breaths and to wait five seconds before she took in
> another breath. After just a few minutes of this simple, delib-
> erate technique, she was able to let go of the gripping tension
> she held with her pain.

Conscious Breathing

The immediate effects of conscious breathing are well illustrated
here. Conscious breathing immediately relaxes our muscles, releases tension, and gives us a feeling of well-being. This is why
deep breathing is so critical in childbirth, helping mom remain
calm, relaxed, and focused.

Anyone who smokes will tell you a cigarette helps calm
them down when they're feeling stressed. Aside from the psy-

chological effect, it's really not the cigarette that helps them relax since nicotine is a stimulant, it's the deep breath they take in when they drag on the cigarette. Unfortunately, they are also breathing in hundreds of harmful chemicals from that cigarette smoke. For my clients who are trying to quit smoking, learning conscious breathing techniques is a major part of their smoking cessation program.

Conscious breathing techniques help us increase our lung capacity and increase our energy. How deeply we breathe directly affects our stress levels, our ability to think clearly, and even our vital signs. We can regulate our heart rate and blood pressure by consciously changing the rhythm and depth of our breathing. This phenomenon is the whole premise behind biofeedback.

The benefits of conscious breathing can be gradual and sometimes go unnoticed. It increases stamina, improves speech and voice, and enhances sleeping patterns. It took me a long time to figure out my feelings of renewal and well-being after my yoga practice are not merely due to the postures I do. Those feelings come from my conscious breathing that is required to perform the postures.

Taking in my breath more consciously, deeply, and slowly allows me to take in my life more consciously, deeply, and slowly. When I don't practice yoga and conscious breathing, I notice the difference. I feel more closed down, more resistant, and less focused.

When we live life like an emergency, when our lives are spinning out of control and we are feeling overwhelmed, we tend to push full speed ahead, going even faster. We may have tension headaches, upset stomachs, and sleepless nights. Instead of taking a pill, what we really need to do is stop, take a pause, and practice conscious breathing. This keeps us present and permits our bodies to relax, our minds to quiet, and our awareness to peak.

> Susan had suffered with severe asthma since she was a young girl. She had recently lost her job, which forced her to move back in with her parents. She was very anxious about her current situation and struggled with chronic respiratory infections and sleepless nights. Susan came to see me for stress management.
>
> The first time I met Susan, I observed her rapid and shallow breathing. Like most of us, she needed to learn how to breathe consciously. We practiced some breathing techniques together and I instructed her to do them on her own for at least five minutes, twice a day and whenever she began to feel anxious.
>
> Two weeks later when Susan came back to see me, she looked like a different person. Her breathing rate had slowed down significantly and her facial expression and body language appeared more relaxed. She told me she felt less anxious when she remembered to breathe consciously. By taking in more breath, Susan was taking in more life.

Learning the Basics

Conscious breathing is a skill that requires practice. There are numerous breathing techniques to help facilitate your conscious breathing. I highly recommend taking a yoga or meditation class for further instruction. For even more intensive training, there are therapists who specialize in teaching effective breathing methods. Use these basic guidelines to get you started:

○ Choose a hard-backed chair or lie on the floor.

○ Wear loose, comfortable clothing.

○ Try inhaling through your nose and exhaling through your mouth.

○ Begin each of these techniques after you have taken a few moments to quiet your mind and settle yourself into a relaxed state.

○ Stay relaxed and calm. Be open to these new experiences of breathing; don't struggle to "do it right."

○ Don't force your breathing or strain to do the exercise.

○ If you become dizzy at any time during the practice, you are probably overexerting yourself. Take a break, relax, and slowly try again.

Witnessing Your Breath

Become aware of your breathing by closing your eyes and focusing on your breath without changing or judging it. Notice your inhalation and your exhalation.

Give yourself a few rounds of breathing to explore each of the questions below. Try to breathe normally without changing it while you witness it. Your goal is to increase your awareness of your natural breathing pattern, not make a judgment about it.

○ **Location:** Place one hand on your lower belly and one hand on your breastbone at the center of your chest. Where do you notice the movement of your breath most: in the lower part or the upper part of your body?

○ **Origin:** Where does the movement of your breath begin?

○ **Frequency:** How fast or slow is your breath? Count your breaths for one minute. Twelve to fourteen breaths per minute is considered an average rate.

○ **Phrasing:** Is there any difference between the length of your inhalation and the length of your exhalation? Are they equal?

○ **Texture:** Is the texture of your breath smooth and even or jerky and uneven?

○ **Depth:** Does your breath feel deep or shallow?

○ **Quality:** What words would you use to describe the quality of your breath? Labored? Easy? Raspy? Quiet?

Continue to focus on your breathing for the next five minutes. As your mind wanders, gently bring your attention back to your breath. To keep focused on your breath, count your inhalations up to ten, and then back down to one and continue this for five minutes.

Breathing Techniques

Once you become aware of your own natural breathing patterns, try these three different breathing styles. See which one feels most comfortable for you.

Diaphragmatic Breathing (Abdominal Breathing)

One of the reasons most of us breathe shallow is because we are more concerned about having flat bellies than taking in full, deep breaths. To take in a full breath, we have to relax our bellies, which relaxes our diaphragm, an important muscle in breathing.

As you inhale, place your hands on your abdomen. Imagine your belly is a balloon, expanding as it relaxes and fills with air. As your belly fills up, your back will arch slightly. As you exhale, your balloon deflates, your belly becomes more flat, and your back presses into your chair or the floor. Do several rounds of this slow, full diaphragmatic breathing.

The Lengthening Breath

We generally focus on taking in full, deep breaths to improve our *inhalation* when we think of improving our breathing. But exhaling is the equally important second half of the breathing cycle. By lengthening our exhalation, we allow the inhalation to also lengthen.

After you witness a few rounds of inhalations and exhalations, see if you can lengthen your exhalation slightly, just for a second or two. Invite your exhalations to be deeper and longer, without straining or becoming uncomfortable. Your inhalations will naturally deepen when your exhalations deepen. Do this for several rounds of breathing and notice the relaxation effect of lengthening your exhalations.

The Three-Part Breath

When we breathe shallow, we tend to use only the upper part of our lungs. This exercise will help you utilize more of your entire lung capacity.

Visually divide the trunk of your body into three parts for breathing. Your abdomen below your bellybutton is the first part, your mid-torso above your bellybutton is the second, and your upper chest is the third. Imagine your breath moving like a wave throughout the three different parts of your trunk. As you inhale, visualize first filling up your lower abdomen by expanding your stomach, then your mid-torso, then your upper chest. As you exhale, empty the air out in the reverse order: your upper chest first your mid-torso next, and your lower abdomen last. Do this for the next few minutes and notice how it feels to use your full lung capacity.

[Your Care Plan]

1 Experiment with each of the breathing techniques by taking your time and allowing five to ten minutes for each one. Select the one that feels most comfortable to you and think about how you could incorporate it into your daily life. You can practice conscious breathing any time you think of it—in

your car, waiting for appointments, watching TV, even first thing in the morning, before you start your day. Just a few minutes of conscious breathing practice on a daily basis will help you incorporate it into your natural breathing patterns.

2 When you feel stressed or anxious, you are probably either holding your breath or breathing too fast and shallow (hyperventilating). The next time you feel stressed, practice a conscious breathing technique just for a few minutes and see if it helps to calm or relax you. Place a "breathe" sign someplace in your view all day to help remind you.

3 Consider taking a class in yoga or meditation to assist you in your practice of conscious breathing. Remain open to all of the possibilities when you choose to consciously breathe in more life.

Chapter 5

Changing Status

"Life is change"
—The Dalai Lama

Change is inevitable. Nothing ever stays the same in our everyday lives, even if we want it to. We move on, grow up, and make decisions that keep us in a constant changing status. When we make ourselves aware of the changes going on, and anticipate that situations may change, we can make the necessary adaptations and adjustments, because when *anything* in our life changes, *everything* in our life changes.

We all know major life-changing events in our lives are very stressful, like getting married, getting divorced, or the death of someone close to us. But the small changes—seemingly minor alterations and adjustments in our lives—can be surprisingly significant. We may not recognize these "adjustments" as changes because we often don't realize how significant they are. The cumulative effects of these smaller things need to be acknowledged because they are indeed life changing.

Recognize and Acknowledge Change

The first step in dealing with change effectively is to recognize it for what it is. When I first see a new lifestyle counseling client,

I ask them if they've had any recent changes in their lives. Many respond "No, not really" at first, but when we dig a little deeper and explore their day-to-day activities, we uncover events that they weren't recognizing as changes in their lives. What follows is a list of life changes that I've found to be the most significant and the least understood and appreciated by my clients.

Professional
Promotion or demotion

Organizational chart change

Fired or hired someone

Job position or job description changed

Shift or schedule changed

Job felt more busy or more stressful

Cutbacks or layoffs

Forced overtime

Conflict with boss or coworker(s)

More frustrated or discouraged with position

More challenged in position

Personal
Acquired a new roommate, a new pet, or a new family
    member to share home

Remodeled home

Moved, bought, or sold home

Less sleep

Change in health

Less energy or any other physical limitation

Felt depressed, lonely, or bored

Eating habits changed

Faith or spirituality changed

Daily routine changed

Started or stopped a medication

Started or stopped an addictive behavior like smoking or drinking caffeine

Family

Kids started school (college or kindergarten)

Family member was ill

Someone close died

Spouse or child went through a difficult time

Supported a family member emotionally or financially

Extra family obligations

More family visits

Social

New activity added (yoga, exercise, art class, etc.)

Joined a new committee, association, or club

Took on a new responsibility for a group

Developed a new relationship (romantic or platonic)

A close friend or family member married or divorced

A close friend or family member moved away

Financial

Income increased or decreased significantly

One significant financial decision made

Unexpected large bill
Windfall of money
Focused on my money more

Because life is change, it is crucial for us to be aware of it.
And if we are not aware of something, we cannot acknowledge
it. When we try to keep our same schedules, our same behaviors, and our same expectations in the face of change, we end up
living life like an emergency! Acknowledging change gives us the
awareness we need to move forward and make the appropriate
adjustments.

Anticipate Change

When we learn how to recognize the changes in our lives, we
can more easily anticipate them. Anticipating change in the ER
is a critical skill. The unstable ER patient's status always changes
either by improving or deteriorating. Treatment priorities change
when the patient's status changes, so it critical that ER staff be
able to predict and respond to changes immediately.

> An anxious-looking man carried his twenty-four-year-old wife
> into the ER. She was very pale and weak after experiencing a
> grueling home birth. After laboring for over forty-eight hours,
> she delivered a healthy baby girl, but had still not delivered the
> placenta, which normally delivers within twenty minutes after
> the baby. Her husband brought her in when she started
> talking nonsense and couldn't even stand up on her own.

The nurse anticipated this woman was in trouble because of her pasty color and her fast heart rate. She called the OB surgeon immediately. After being in the treatment room for less than five minutes, the patient lost consciousness. Her breathing became shallow and her blood pressure dropped to almost nothing.

Fortunately, the OB surgeon was on his way and took her to surgery immediately to remove the remaining placenta that caused her to hemorrhage. Although she required many transfusions to replace all the blood she lost, she was very fortunate, because she would have bled to death had she not been taken to surgery.

This woman was not capable of anticipating her status change, but thankfully her husband and nurse did. If her husband hadn't noticed her change in coherency and weakness and insisted on bringing her to the ER, and if the nurse had not foreseen the critical situation, this young mother would not have survived.

Sometimes even the most obvious of changes escape us in our own lives. When we can anticipate change, we can prepare for it and make the transitions with more ease. We can also save ourselves a lot of the frustration and turmoil when it catches us by surprise.

My husband and I moved to a small mountain town a few years ago, sixty minutes from the familiar metropolitan area I had lived in for years. After the move, I struggled to keep my work schedule, routines, and social commitments the same. I quickly became very frustrated and resentful, driving up and down the canyon every day, instead of enjoying my new mountain home.

What was I thinking? I couldn't possibly keep my same life if I was living in a different location sixty miles away. If I would have anticipated this major change in my life better, and immediately sought the necessary resources such as a hairdresser, a doctor, a yoga center, and new social circles, I would have transitioned into my new community much easier.

Embrace Change

Once we recognize and anticipate change, we start to embrace it. Many of the changes we experience in our lives are difficult because even though we gain something, we also lose something. We don't always consider the losses involved with a new job, combining households, or having a baby. The loss of freedom, time, and familiarity is significant and needs to be embraced when we monitor our life for change.

Our culture does not support many of the changes we experience in life, especially the inevitable process of aging. Movie stars keep our expectations unrealistic by getting tucked, trimmed, and lifted with cosmetic surgery. We treat menopause—a normal season of a woman's life—like a terminal illness, promoting all kinds of remedies to help women "get through it." Instead of honoring aging and the wisdom and enrichment that it offers, we spend enormous amounts of time and money trying to avoid it.

Embracing change requires us to adjust the way we look at things and how we value them. This often requires us to shift our priorities and make some difficult decisions. When we try to keep everything the same, even in the midst of major life-changing events, we are trying to avoid the discomfort that accompanies change. When we use this avoidance technique and don't accept it, we end up struggling with the change even more.

> Sally was an exceptional ER physician. I met her just after she finished residency and had her first child. A year later, she had a second one, and returned to work six weeks after her delivery. Now with two young daughters, Sally was burdened with conflicting emotions, feeling guilty about her children when she was at work and feeling exhausted from working when she was with them at home.
>
> After several months of struggling with her schedule and feeling like she was never doing the right thing, Sally gave up medicine to be a full-time stay-at-home mom. It was a difficult decision for her to make because not only did it affect her family financially, it also forced Sally to examine her priorities and sense of self-worth.
>
> Not everyone was supportive of her life-changing decision, and friends and family asked, "How could you give up medicine after all that hard work and so many years of school?" Sally thoughtfully replied, "Being a physician was the only thing I thought I ever wanted, but I realized being a mom was something I wanted even more."

Embracing change is not always easy. We have to accept the fact that as our life circumstances change, our priorities have to change. We have to be willing to go through the discomfort of both losing and gaining something, and we have to change our expectations of ourselves and everyone else.

How can I embrace change?

—————————— [R$_x$] ——————————

- ▫ Change your perspective from *if* things change to *when* things change.
- ▫ Accept that "life is change" and value the growth, enrichment, and wisdom it provides.
- ▫ Welcome the opportunity to learn flexibility, compassion, and resiliency with change.
- ▫ Recognize that change gives you appreciation for the right here, right now, instead of taking it for granted.
- ▫ Allow yourself a transition period when things change, a time for grieving, reflection, and adjustment.
- ▫ Make the necessary adjustments in your behaviors and your expectations with a change

[Your Care Plan]

1 Take an inventory of your life changes by circling all the appropriate statements in the lists on page 52–54 that apply to you within the last three to six months. Make a list of any additional changes not mentioned already.

If you circled more than three life changes for the last three to six months, you probably need to make some adjustments in your expectations and your behaviors. Remember that when you add in a new commitment or responsibility, you have to take something out to make room for it. For example, if you started taking an art class one night a week, then you might have to give up going to the gym that same day. If you suffer a loss of any kind, you need to replace it with something else. When you quit smoking, you have to replace the old familiar behavior with a new one, like taking a short walk outside when you normally would be taking a smoking break.

2 Consider the following questions:

Are you surprised by how many changes you checked for the last few months?

Do you have a better understanding of why things "just don't seem the same?"

Are you having any unrealistic expectations of yourself or others?

Is there anything you have been struggling with to keep the same?

Do you need to shift any behaviors in your daily routine?

Do you need to reconsider any of your priorities?

3 How could you embrace a change going on in your life right now instead of resisting it?

Example:

My work schedule is changing and I will be working opposite hours from my husband's schedule. I can embrace this change by relishing my time alone and doing things I wouldn't ordinarily have the opportunity to do.

Chapter 6

The Treatment Plan

"Intention is the power of the experience."
—Cynthia Gale

For every diagnosis, from a heart attack to an ankle sprain, there is a specific treatment plan to manage the problem and care for the patient. Once the patient is assessed and the diagnosis is determined, the treatment plan is initiated. This plan is specific to the diagnosis and provides deliberate and calculated diagnostic tests, medications, and procedures to address the patient's problems.

Treatment plans are very intentional. They have been tried, tested, and found successful. Treatment plans consistently and efficiently provide the patient the best care available. In this way, every health care provider will treat a specific diagnosis, such as dehydration, based on the treatment plan and certain patient criteria, not on the day of the week, or what they might whimsically feel like doing that day.

If we didn't use a specific treatment plan in the ER, patient care would be unpredictable, unreliable, and unsafe. We would never know for sure if the treatment would work because it would always be a test, an experiment, a good guess. Is that how you want to live your life?

Just like the treatment plan in the ER, we need a personal plan to manage our everyday lives. This plan is our intention, our purpose, and, most importantly, our choice. When we choose to live with intention, we recognize our purpose for doing what we do and being where we are.

In a Colorado mountain-town ER where I worked for many years, the number one summer diagnosis was dehydration. Our summers are hot and dry, and visitors often forgot how much more water they needed to drink to make up for the high altitude, even though they "didn't sweat." Whether we saw healthy young men turn weak as kittens or little old ladies suffer "fainting spells," the treatment plan for dehydration was fairly routine and very specific.

A large, muscular twenty-three-year-old man was practically carried in by his buddy as he weakly mumbled, "I'm really sick." The two were camping and had spent the last three days hiking in the nearby National Park. The patient complained of nausea and vomiting, diarrhea, abdominal pain, and generalized weakness—all classic signs of dehydration.

The treatment plan for dehydration was initiated. After baseline vital signs were taken, blood work was sent to the lab and an IV was inserted to provide replacement fluids. Medication for nausea and vomiting was also given.

This patient required several bags of IV fluids before his vital signs returned to normal and he urinated, both signs of rehydration. It is common to have to replace three or four liters of fluid, but he had seven liters before he could urinate! We sent him back to his camp several hours later rehydrated and feeling much better. The treatment plan was successful.

Living with Intention

Intentional living, like the treatment plan, is about being mindful, being present, and being deliberate in our thoughts and our actions. Without intention we have no path, no plan, and no way to gauge if we are doing it right. We may never feel like we are in the right place at the right time. My clients will say, "When I'm at work all I can think about is being home and when I'm home I constantly think about work." This internal struggle keeps them always second-guessing themselves.

When we choose to live with intention, we have more confidence and control in our lives. We are the ones choosing what to do and how to be. And even more important, we know *why* we do what we do, which is immensely satisfying and self-enriching. Being in control and choosing our own direction keeps us on track with ourselves and our lives.

Living with intention requires us to be present to the moment. Staying conscious and present when we are doing anything or doing nothing—like stopping (see Chapter 3)—can be challenging and requires both discipline and practice. A friend of mine who has been active in Alcoholics Anonymous for years says it well: *"You can't stay sober if you can't stay conscious."*

We often go to extremes not to be intentional. We overeat, drink too much alcohol, and spend lots of money to escape, numb out, and not be conscious. One of my clients told me she is "consciously unconscious" about her eating when she wants to numb out and not be responsible for it. Being intentional requires you to take responsibility for where you are and what you are doing in your life. It requires you to feel and experience, even when you don't want to.

Walk, Don't Run

Our society is one of multitasking. We always have so much to do, we think we are better off if we can do more than one thing at a time, and even better if we can do it quickly. Living with intention is walking instead of running through our lives. Walking allows us to feel, taste, and live each experience fully and consciously.

Unfortunately, our culture doesn't always support this and we often focus on making the experience high-producing and efficient. But is it, really?

I was having lunch with a good friend at an upscale Italian restaurant when two well-dressed men sat down at the table next to us. During their entire meal, they both talked on their cell phones, in separate conversations. I wondered why they bothered to go out for lunch. They could have just as well stayed at their desks, because they weren't going to remember what they ate for lunch and with whom they ate it anyway.

Choose Intention

Intention is a choice, not a "should." Living with intention must be simple and light or we make too many rules for ourselves and get caught up in all of those "shoulds." No decision ends up being a decision when we "should" on ourselves, like this:

"I am so tired today, but I really should get some work done."

"I am feeling lonely today, but I should buck up and stay home anyway."

"I really don't want to go tonight, but I should because I said I would."

"I should have gotten more done today."

There are many ways we can practice being intentional. After years of attempting it, I finally realize the many benefits of yoga, including how it helps me be present to the moment. Throughout the entire class my yoga teacher reminds us to stay aware of our bodies, our minds, and our breath. My mind used to wander off, making lists, planning meals, and solving all my problems. Now I can gently bring myself back to the present and am grateful for this opportunity to practice being intentional. My early morning yoga practice helps me remain more conscious and present throughout the day.

We can choose to be intentional in all of our activities. Going to a meditation class can offer inner peace and solace or fellowship. Attending a national convention can be a professional obligation or a networking opportunity. When we choose *why* we do what we do, we live with intention.

It is interesting to observe the different intentions of people who go to the same place, like my local health club. The time of day they go, the clothing they wear, and what they do when they get there are all part of their intention. Whether it is socializing, bodybuilding, or good old-fashioned sweating, the intentions can be unique to each person.

I strive to remain open but to set an intention for anything I do, whether it is going to the gym or staying at home in my pajamas. My needs vary depending on my mood and different times during the day. I may want distraction, full involvement, or just quiet time to myself. What we choose our intention to be is not nearly as important as the fact that we actively choose it.

At the Women's Mountain Retreats I facilitate (see Chapter 12), we always begin the retreat by setting our intentions for the weekend. Each woman comes with different needs, and by actively identifying them she can make the appropriate choices to meet those needs and plan her weekend retreat accordingly.

But when things don't go exactly as planned—and often they don't—we need to be flexible with our intentions, and remain open to the outcome and not attached to our original expectations. Have you ever had something not turn out exactly as you planned? Sometimes, that can be a blessing.

Harriet was dreading the Women's Mountain Retreat. She was sponsored by her workplace and that was the only reason she was going. She didn't have time for this; she had so much to do at home, and work was piling up at her second job. She had already decided to sneak out early on Sunday.

After dinner that first evening, Harriet felt quite different once she had met the other women at the retreat. As they all shared their concerns and fears, Harriet discovered she had a lot in common with them. She ended up staying for the entire weekend, and made some significant life decisions during the retreat.

Harriet decided to quit her second job and postpone going back to school. She also connected with a woman she still keeps in contact with today.

Harriet's initial intention was to just to "get through" the weekend. But she remained open to the outcome and ended up getting so much more from the retreat than she'd expected.

How can I live with intention?

——————— [Rx] ———————

☐ Be deliberate with your everyday activities as well as special events. Know why are you going, what you want, and what you need from the experience.

☐ Write about your purpose for doing things before your day begins, and reflect on it at the day's end.

☐ Trust that you are exactly where you are supposed to be, and stand in the space you are in by being present to the moment, not always trying to "get there."

☐ Remain open. Keep your intentions simple and flexible and don't get bogged down with "shoulding" on yourself.

[Your Care Plan]

1 Today, practice being present to the moment by being conscious and mindful of one activity you do. The more mundane or boring it is, the better. This is for you to practice being in the moment.

Consciously choose to do this one thing at a time and to really focus on this one thing, like doing the dishes. Notice how the warm water feels, how slippery the plate is when you start, and how squeaky clean it is after you wash it.

Avoid obvious distractions to your intentional activity such as talking on the phone, the TV, or loud music.

Whatever activity you decide to do, try doing it slower.

While you practice being in the moment with your activity, consciously bring back your wandering or busy mind to the present.

2 Upon waking, ask yourself the following questions about your approaching day. While these may seem basic and obvious questions, they need to be addressed in order to set your intention.

What do I need today?

Example: I need to connect with someone I trust

_____

What do I see as the most important event of the day for me?

Meeting my best friend for lunch

_____

What am I most concerned or anxious about today?

The sales presentation I will give

_____

_____

What do I need to do to lessen my anxiety and feel better about it?

Rehearse my program this morning

What am I most excited about today?

Meeting my best friend for lunch

What will it take to make this a "good day" for me?

A good workout
Knowing I have done my best at the sales presentation
Feeling I am heard and supported by my best friend

After answering these questions, set your intention so that you will get your needs met today.

When setting your intentions, be very clear and specific. Start out by writing just one. Write it on an index card, a sticky note, or a small piece of paper to have in your view the whole day.

Example: Today, my intention is: To connect with my best friend and get the support I need.

---

3 Pick a whole day for your personal treatment plan and schedule it in your calendar right now. Now create a totally intentional experience that will nurture your body, mind, and

spirit both physically and emotionally. Start with waking up and end with going to sleep.

What do you do? Where do you go? Who are you with?

Do you spend four hours in your favorite bookstore?

Do you take a bath? Do you take a nap?

What do you eat?

Where are you drawn to?

Is your intention to be laid back and see what the day brings, or do you have a lot of structure and appointments?

Remember, this is your personal treatment plan based on what your needs are *that day*.

Feel free to fantasize and be wild with your intentions, then reel yourself back in and make a realistic plan. Your intention can change as your mood and needs change, so remain flexible and open.

Example:

My intention:

Rest and connect with some important people in my life.

Wake up on my own without an alarm

Practice yoga

Meditate

Walk to my favorite coffee shop and leisurely read the paper

Take a gentle hike with my dog

Meet my best friend for sushi

Browse through the bookstore

Get a massage

Take a long, hot bath with aromatherapy

Have a candlelight dinner with my husband (prepared by him)

Snuggle with my husband in front of the fire and watch a romantic comedy

Go to bed whenever I feel like it

_____

_____

_____

_____

_____

_____

_____

_____

4 After you have lived your intentional day, write about what it was like. What did you really enjoy? What made you feel really special? How could you incorporate some part of it into your life every day, or even every week?

_____

_____

_____

_____

_____

_____

_____

Chapter 7
The Overdose

"Life has a practice of living you if you don't live it."
–Philip Larkin

*O*verdosing is *overdoing,* overindulging, or getting too much of anything in our everyday lives to our own detriment. Whether it is rich food, aerobic exercise, or holiday parties, we can get too much of a good thing. Unlike what many of us have come to believe, in a culture where we supersize everything, more is not always better.

Today we have bigger houses, fuller schedules, and more opportunities to overdo than ever before. We are busy, we are frantic, and we are too much! And we still continue to ask ourselves, "how can I get more done?"

An overdose in the ER is the patient who has ingested too much of something, either intentionally or accidentally: too much medication, too many beers, or too much of any recreational drug. Because the treatment plan for overdoses can vary according to quantity and composition of the substance, the ER nurse must find out what the substance was, how much was taken, and when it was ingested. In most overdose circumstances, unfortunately, the patient isn't able to communicate this critical information.

I saw a small, female figure at the end of the corridor hanging on to a wall, moaning something I couldn't understand. I raced down the hall and by the time I reached her, she had fallen to the floor, unresponsive. I yelled for help, and several staff members carefully lifted her limp body onto a stretcher and rolled her into the ER.

The team moved quickly to check her vital signs, assess her respirations, and prepare to place a tube in her throat to help her breathe. Not knowing why this patient was unconscious, I searched her purse for any helpful medical information. She was thirty-four years old and had two sons, who looked to be about six and eight years old from their baseball pictures.

I also found several empty prescription bottles for antidepressants and sleeping pills. She would now be treated as a suspected drug overdose. The team prepared to pump out her stomach, a messy procedure that removes all of the stomach contents, including any medications ingested.

This young woman later insisted her drug overdose was not intentional. Her long history of depression had been exacerbated by a painful divorce. She wasn't sleeping well and took more antidepressants than prescribed because she "just wanted to feel better."

We can overdo virtually anything in our day-to-day lives to try to feel better. In my Lifestyle Counseling practice, I observe five key areas my clients consistently overdo: 1) food intake, 2) exercise, 3) work responsibilities, 4) social life, and 5) spending.

Food Intake

We all have overindulged on food at one time or another. Eating too much dressing and pumpkin pie at Thanksgiving is accepted, expected, and even encouraged in our society. But we also overdo our sugar intake for that instant sugar buzz, caffeine consumption to jump-start us, and high-fat foods to give us comfort.

We overdo our food intake to feed our emotional needs, not our physical ones. When we overdo our eating, we are not necessarily overhungry. More likely we are overtired, bored, or stressed.

Exercise

Overdoing our exercise can be tied to overindulging in food. Some people even use exercise as a way to purge the excess calories they have eaten. If more is better, then 60 minutes must be better than 30 minutes, and 90 is better yet.

I have a tendency to overexercise because it relieves my stress and releases those great endorphins. But when I exercise to the point of hurting myself and continue to exercise even when I suffer overuse injuries, I am overdoing it. Your body has a great way of getting your attention when you overdo it at the gym if you only listen to it.

Work

If you are overdoing your work, there is no way you can have a healthy family life or take time for yourself. With today's work ethic, where we are all expected to do more with less, your company will try to squeeze everything out of you they can. If you skip lunch and work late every day, there probably won't be anyone to chastise you on your overdoing, unless maybe your spouse.

We have to value ourselves for who we are, and not just what we do. The downside of overdoing your work is that you create unrealistic expectations of what you can accomplish for both yourself and your superiors. We all have crunch times when more is expected of us, but if you consistently skip lunch, stay late, and take work home on the weekends trying to get it all done, you are overdoing your work. Richard Carlson from *Don't Sweat the Small Stuff* tells us our inbox isn't *supposed* to be empty. This is job security!

Social Life

Can we really party too much? Of course we can. You know how most of us feel by January, going to more holiday parties in three weeks' time than we do the entire year. Even really fun parties aren't fun anymore if we get too much of them.

I know some people who seem to know everyone and go everywhere, but they can never really stay very long because they're always moving on to the next thing. One year, I was invited to three parties in one evening. Instead of choosing which one to go to, I went to all three, and really didn't go to any of them. I now know to go deep instead of wide in my social circles and to accept a select few invitations. This allows me to be present and really enjoy the things I choose to say yes to.

My single clients say they are afraid their friends might stop calling if they don't go out every time they're invited. If someone says to you, "It's been so long since we got together, I guess you don't have time for me anymore," listen carefully. They may be right.

Spending

"Retail therapy" can be a good thing to do for yourself occasionally. But if you are hauling to the mall every time you feel bad or—even worse—gotten yourself involved in the Home Shopping Network, beware! The way our credit cards give us instant cash these days, it is very easy to get into a lot of debt—fast.

Besides realizing that a great cashmere sweater on sale will cost us three times as much by the time we pay the interest, we need to look at what needs are being fulfilled with our overspending. I have often thought it would be revealing to go to a mall and interview some of the women shopping there, especially when I see them making large and impulsive purchases. I don't think the retailers would be too supportive of me, but it would be a fascinating study.

Crooked Coping Mechanisms

Overdoing contributes to emergency living because we are trying to do too much. But the truth is, we just can't overdo everything in our life; there (thankfully) just isn't enough time. But when we overdo one thing or one area, it becomes a "crooked coping mechanism. " It is crooked because it creates an imbalance when we neglect some aspect of our lives while we overdo another. So often we overdo in one area of our lives to distract us from issues or activities we want to avoid.

In order to live a balanced life, to live fully, we have to address all areas of our lives—our work, our relationships, and our own self-care.

Carol is a bright, attractive woman. She loved her job and, at thirty-eight, had successfully climbed the corporate ladder of a small software company. When she came to see me, Carol was approximately seventy-five pounds overweight. Carol's physician had referred her to me for some health issues affected by her weight.

Carol quickly admitted her life revolved around work, and she spent sixty to seventy hours a week at the office. She was working so much that she neglected relationships, exercise, and her own self-care. Carol felt uncomfortable in social situations because of her extra weight, and ended up "feeding" her loneliness with high-calorie snack foods.

Carol knew she was in a rut. Overdoing her work life kept her safe, but it also kept her stuck feeling lonely and unhappy. When she got sick and tired of being sick and tired of her life, she made some significant changes.

Cutting back on her work hours allowed Carol the time and energy to join a gym. After she lost some weight, she felt better physically and started to regain her self-confidence in social situations. Carol learned how to balance her life with her exercise, social activities, and work, without overdoing any of them.

Why Overdose?

Just like the ER patient, we can overdo our lives intentionally or accidentally, but there is always a reason, even if it is subconscious. We tend to overdo things in our lives for one of three reasons: We want what is familiar and comfortable, we want immediate pleasure, or we want to feel like we are enough.

We can easily overdo those things that are comfortable and familiar to us. If we are overdoing our work, it's probably because we are pretty good at it. When we overdo, we are overcompensating for an area we may not feel as confident in or as comfortable with, as when Carol was overdoing her work and neglecting her social life.

We also think we'll feel better if we overdo something. If I am bored and eat a huge piece of chocolate cake at 2 in the afternoon, I may feel better after the first bite, but after I finish the whole piece, I feel guilty and my stomach is upset. The pleasure is very short-lived and now I am miserable.

Finally, we may overdo areas in our lives just because we think we *should* do more in order to "be enough." Feeling like we are not enough is our own perception and we will overdo and give 150 percent instead of the 100 percent to compensate for it. We need to find our own sense of worth and value not in what we do, but in who we are. This is a difficult concept to grasp, and requires us to make a major shift in our thinking and feelings of self-worth.

We don't usually judge others by how much they do or how much they get accomplished. We value our friends, our coworkers, our family members for *who* they are, whether they be curious, congruent, funny, or loyal. These are probably the same traits we admire in ourselves. We can make the shift in our "not enough" thinking by focusing on these positive traits, on who we are, instead of what we do. An interesting exercise is one where you ask five people who know you well to describe who you are, not what you do. In other words, not a good mother or experienced nurse but loving, generous, or bright. This will help you shift your focus on appreciating who you are, instead of what you do.

Without making this shift, we will always look for the next thing to accomplish and fulfill us. And we will never be enough to fulfill ourselves until we can accept that we are valid and valuable for who we are.

Too Much

Are you too much? Are you trying to be or do too much? Are you overdosing? It's not always easy to determine when and how the shift of doing too much to being enough needs to take place, but we don't have to start with major life decisions. We can start out small and learn by contrast, catching ourselves overdoing and remembering that lesson the next time. I cannot always predict if I will overdo something beforehand, and I sure can't detect it while I'm doing it, but I clearly see it afterwards, and so does everyone else.

> I was really tired even before I made the two-hour drive to my monthly association meeting. I got up at 5:00 a.m. on a Saturday to be there by 8:00 a.m.

I left the meeting promptly at noon, without eating lunch, because I had "so much to do." I made the grave mistake of attempting several errands on the Saturday afternoon of a holiday weekend. I found no place to park, long lines, and everyone else impatient and in a hurry, just like me.

It took me almost three hours to drive home in the heavy holiday traffic. When I finally arrived, I was exhausted, hungry, and grouchy. I immediately started yelling at my husband, asking him, "What have you done all day?" His standard answer of "Not much" infuriated me!

Afterwards, I realized how ridiculous it was for me to be mad at him just because I had done too much and I thought he hadn't done enough. Thankfully, being the wiser one of us, he put me to bed and ignored my ranting and raving.

We must determine for ourselves how much is too much because we all have different energy levels and thresholds for activity. A successful retired banker once told me he liked to have just a little more to do than he could handle, to keep him on his toes. My husband, on the other hand, requires lots of downtime to recharge his batteries and keep him on his toes.

Am I overdoing my life?

——————— **[Rx]** ———————

You are if you:

☐ feel run-down or tired more often than not.

- experience overuse injuries to your back, neck, knees, or ankles.
- feel resentful for always being "the one."
- have people tell you, "I know you're really busy, but…"
- are " accident-prone" in your car, in the kitchen, or anywhere else.
- forget an appointment, a date, or a celebration.
- don't even consider if something might be too much to take on.
- always look ahead for the next thing to get done.
- value yourself for what you do, not who you are.
- know there are areas in your life right now you are neglecting.

Overdone Holidays

The holidays offer a great opportunity for us to overdo because we cram more spending, baking, and partying into two months than in the rest of the year. A lot of us have issues that come up during the holidays, but instead of facing them, we keep ourselves busy, stressed, and distracted. With our schedules already overextended and demanding, it's no wonder so many people equate the holidays with exhaustion, disappointment, and "jingle bills."

How can I avoid overdoing the holidays?

———————— [R$_x$] ————————

- **Remember what you love.**
  Think about what brings you true joy during the

holidays. Continue doing what you like to do, and let
go of the things you don't. I gave up sending cards
many years ago, but I still love to decorate and
entertain.

- **Be open to new family traditions.**
  Sometimes we get in a rut with our traditions. It
  doesn't always have to be the same way every year, so
  experiment and see how you can simplify the holiday
  by doing it differently.

- **Budget your time and money.**
  Decide how much time and money you can honestly
  spend on the holidays, and keep to your budget.

- **Avoid malls, the kitchen, and airports.**
  If a crowded mall gives you as much anxiety as a root
  canal, rely on catalogs and on-line shopping. If you
  love to cook, by all means go for it, but if you feel like
  an unappreciated slave all day, consider catering big
  meals or going out. If traveling during the holiday
  stresses you out, stay home and visit faraway family at
  a less hectic time.

[Your Care Plan]

Are you too much? Being aware of what we are overdoing is the
first step to changing it. This is an awareness exercise to help you
closely examine the five areas I consistently see my clients overdoing: eating, exercise, work responsibilities, relationships, and
spending. Check the statements that apply to you.

Food Intake
___I eat sugar at least once a day.

___I drink more than one alcoholic beverage a day.

___I drink caffeine to get me going in the morning and keep me going in the afternoon.

___I eat in front of the TV.

___I eat ice cream, peanut butter, and cheese for comfort.

___I eat when I am not stomach-hungry, but mouth-hungry.

___I don't allow myself to get hungry.

___I can eat something that tastes good until I feel sick.

___I wake up in the morning full.

___I get nervous if I start feeling empty.

Exercise

___When I overeat, I make up for it by overexercising.

___I consistently spend more than one hour a day at the gym.

___The only way I know how to manage my stress is with a good workout.

___If I don't really push it, I don't feel I am really working out.

___I have had many overuse injuries.

___I have exercised with an injury, pushing through the pain.

___I have exercised when I had a fever.

___My exercise takes precedence over everything else—everything.

___I get worried if I miss a day of exercise.

___I have a hard time taking a day off from my exercise.

Work Responsibilities

___I eat lunch at my desk.

___I work late more than once a week.

___I bring work home with me at night and on the weekend.

___I go in on my days off.

___I always have extra vacation time left at the end of the year.

___I value myself by how much I can get done in a day.

___People have said to me, "You work too much."

___I feel guilty for not spending more time with my family.

___I don't have any hobbies I enjoy.

___I think about my work all the time.

Social Life

___I panic if I don't have my weekend filled with social plans.

___I have trouble being alone.

___I frequently overcommit myself for different events.

___My friends always tell me how busy I am.

___I have a hard time turning down a party, anywhere.

___I'm never home.

___I never want to miss anything.

___I'm afraid if I decline an invitation, I might not be asked again.

Spending

___My credit card bills are more than I can pay off every month.

___I visit a mall at least once a week.

___I purchase something from the Home Shopping Network at least once a week.

___Buying something new for myself always makes me feel better.

___I have purchased many items that I have never worn or used.

___I am attracted to all sales like a magnet.

___I consider myself an impulsive buyer.

___I spend beyond my means.

What other areas are you overdoing that create crooked coping mechanisms? List them here:

_____

_____

_____

_____

_____

_____

Study the items you checked off and the additional list you made. Can you see an overdose? What might you be overcompensating for?

When you overdo in one or more areas, you develop crooked coping mechanisms because there is an imbalance with the things you are not doing. Look at the following list and check anything you feel you are not doing or spending enough time on. When you let go of some of your overdoing, you will be able to address the areas you identify.

Health

___ General health (medications, vitamins, screenings, checkups)

___ Dental health

___ Exercise

___ Eating healthy

___ Drinking water

___ Sleep

___ Rest

Relationships
__Children

__Spouse

__Extended family

__Friendships

__Social activities

__Community

Work
__Networking activities

__Professional organizations

__Parties and celebrations

Play
__Writing

__Cultural events

__Pleasure reading

__Pets

__Sports

__Hobbies

Spirituality
__Church

__Spiritual practices

__Relaxation

__Retreats

Chapter 8
The Adrenaline Junkie

"To see your drama clearly is to be liberated from it."
—Ken Keyes

*L*iving with adrenaline on a daily basis is life-threatening. Many people believe living with chronic stress leads to increased adrenaline. But the truth is, many of us thrive on adrenaline, and this is what leads to chronic stress, or what I call stress exhaustion. Stress exhaustion threatens our health, our relationships, and the quality of our lives. If you are an adrenaline junkie, you also have stress exhaustion in some aspect of your life, because the two are not exclusive.

Adrenaline thrills us and fills us with excitement and exhilaration. Look at the many ways we try to re-create that fear and rush: We watch scary movies, ride roller coasters, and engage in high-risk sports, such as skydiving and car racing. For the short run, adrenaline can serve us well in life-threatening situations, and give us healthy stimulation, but the chronic use of adrenaline leads to stress exhaustion.

Lifesaving Adrenaline
The body's response to stress is to go into a hyperalert state that provides us incredible strength and courage to react in a

life-threatening situation. In life-threatening situations in the ER, where literally seconds count—like when a patient stops breathing, has a fatal heart rhythm, or is bleeding profusely— we call a "code blue" to alert the appropriate personnel for assistance. Everyone drops what they're doing to assist that patient. Everyone knows this is a true emergency, so energy and adrenaline run high, and are necessary to help the staff act quickly and appropriately in these situations.

But it may surprise you to learn these incidents are the exception in the ER, not the rule. For the most part, the ER staff must maintain a controlled and composed environment to remain effective and efficient.

The Adrenaline Junkie

The adrenaline junkie is chronically in a hyperalert state. The flurry of activity they get so used to participating in prevents them from having any composure or real control over themselves in their environment. Look at the way people drive, fight over parking places, or react when someone has too many items in the express lane: They act like they're going to a code blue!

Adrenaline can be destructive to our living when it is released over long periods of time as people become addicted to being in hyperalert and hyperstimulated states. They even create their own "emergency" situations to feed their addiction. They get involved in unhealthy relationships, make unrealistic commitments, and take unnecessary risks, like driving through a snowstorm. As I mentioned in Chapter 1, those of us predisposed to emergency living tend to have a great need for stimulation and adrenaline, and can be referred to as "adrenaline junkies."

Sue thrived on chaos, and the more, the better. Between having three young children, a husband who frequently traveled, and her own job as an emergency medical technician, Sue found plenty of chaos. She operated her life in panic mode, and when there wasn't a crisis at hand, she seemed to create one by taking on another project, signing up for extra overtime, or making a large purchase she couldn't afford.

This stress-producing chaos took its toll on Sue. She developed insomnia and chronic fatigue, and frequently suffered with colds and flu-like symptoms. The final straw was breast cancer. That got her attention.

Sue says breast cancer was the best thing that ever happened to her. "My treatment was exhausting, and I was forced to learn how to conserve my energy. Your perspective really changes when a great day is one when you don't throw up more than three times."

Today, Sue lives a full life with her husband, children, and job, but without all of the chaos and adrenaline.

Am I an adrenaline junkie?

—————————— [Rx] ——————————

You are if you:

- □ are attracted to high-risk activities, such as skydiving or ice climbing.
- □ feel calm and calculated when everyone else is in a panic.
- □ thrive on frenetic activity and go to lengths to create it.

- enjoy the feeling of being charged and wound up.
- require little sleep when you are excited about something.
- grab sugar, caffeine, or anything else to "keep you going."
- always look for the next thing to give you a thrill or rush.
- wait until the last minute to do most things.
- like extremes, including movies, sports, and relationships.
- have difficulty relaxing.

Stress Exhaustion

The chronic use of adrenaline that leads to stress exhaustion is costly. Statistics show stress is a factor in 80 percent of all illnesses, and studies prove that digestive disorders, asthma, diabetes, and depression are just a few of the illnesses exacerbated by stress. Stress exhaustion interrupts our eating and sleeping patterns, depresses our immune system, and even releases more cholesterol into our bloodstream to contribute to heart disease.

When we get so accustomed to living with stress exhaustion, we don't always appreciate the cumulative effect it has on our minds and bodies. In my Lifestyle Counseling practice, one of the first questions I ask my clients is what kind of stress they are dealing with at the moment. Many people don't even realize they are suffering from stress exhaustion, and are always relieved to find out why they feel the way they feel, like having daily headaches, mood swings, or loneliness. Stress exhaustion presents itself with many different symptoms besides the classic change in appetite and difficulty sleeping.

Three symptoms I see a lot in my counseling practice that people often discount are feelings of boredom, apathy, and chronic fatigue. You can see how these can all be related. When we are stressed, we often shut down emotionally and become indifferent to our lives. Apathy certainly leads to boredom: If you can't get excited about anything, you get bored. Apathy and boredom make you feel lethargic and "stuck," which leads to chronic fatigue.... So it becomes a vicious cycle, each symptom feeding off the other. And it all starts with too much adrenaline.

Other symptoms of stress exhaustion are shown in the chart on page 94.

It amazes me how we can disregard even the most major stressful events in our lives. The ER patient frequently fails to mention these events until I ask them a pointed question about the stress going on in their lives.

Working a holiday in the ER is usually very slow or very busy and nothing in between. The patients we treat seem to come in with more problems than usual, ranging from the physical and emotional to the financial and social.

One particularly busy Thanksgiving Day, a mom brought in her thirteen-year-old daughter. They both had the disheveled appearance and aroma of having been in their current clothing for quite some time. The teenager, a known diabetic, came in with continuous vomiting and rapid, labored breathing. She was diagnosed with diabetic ketoacidosis, a serious condition in which blood sugar gets dangerously high. Untreated, it can lead to coma and death. It wasn't until I asked the mother what kind of stress she'd been having in her

Symptoms of Stress Exhaustion

Physical		Spiritual
Accident-prone	Insomnia	Apathy
Change in appetite	Muscle aches	Cynicism
Colds	Nightmares	Doubt
Digestive upsets	Prone to accidents	Emptiness
Fatigue	Rashes	Look for magic
Finger-drumming	Restlessness	Loss of direction
Foot-tapping	Teeth grinding	Loss of meaning
Headaches	Tension	Martyrdom
Heart palpitations	Weight change	Need to prove self
Increased alcohol, drug, tobacco use		Unforgiving

Emotional	Mental	Relational
Anxiety	Boredom	Clamming up
Bad temper	Confusion	Decreased sex drive
Being easily discouraged	Dulled senses	Distrust
Crying spells	Forgetfulness	Hiding
Depression	Lack of creativity	Intolerance
Feeling "no one cares"	Lethargy	Isolation
Frustration	Low productivity	Lack of intimacy
Irritability	Negative attitude	Lashing out
Little joy	Negative self-talk	Less contact w/friends
Mood swings	Poor concentration	Loneliness
Nervous laugh	"Spacing out"	Nagging
Nightmares	Whirling mind	Resentment
"The blues"		Using people
Worrying		

*Based on *Structured Exercises in Stress Management*, Whole Person Press.

life lately that I understood why her daughter's diabetes was out of control.

They were living out of their car in the dead of winter, along with three more children all under the age of ten. They were on the run from mom's estranged husband, who had a history of violent behavior. On a waiting list for the family shelter, they went to the mission every evening for their one meal of the day.

Her family's most basic needs were not being met, so it was understandable that keeping her daughter supplied with insulin was not a priority to mom. As I listened to this woman tell her story with no emotion and no self-pity, I witnessed the numbing effects of stress exhaustion.

Most of us will never experience such stressful conditions in our own lifetime, but we all live with varying degrees of stress. When we are adrenaline junkies and create our own stress exhaustion, the biggest impact we can have on ourselves is to learn how to relax.

Relaxation for the Adrenaline Junkie

So often when someone comes to the ER displaying obvious symptoms of stress, we mechanically say, "Just try to relax." What does that mean to someone in distress? Probably nothing. We have to know *how* to relax before we can *try* to relax. What does relaxation mean to an adrenaline junkie? Usually it means stopping or slowing down, which is very boring. There are some very basic, but not always easy, ways to relax, even if you are an adrenaline junkie.

How do I relax?

———————————— [R$_x$] ————————————

☐ **Practice conscious breathing.**
Take in slow, deep, belly-breaths without forcing or
straining. See if you can lengthen your exhalation, even
for a second or two; this will help you lengthen your
inhalation and relax your mind and body (see Chapter 4).

☐ **Use progressive relaxation.**
Start by tensing the muscles of your face and holding
for ten seconds, then relax your face muscles. Tense
and relax your neck and shoulders, then your arms,
then your abdomen. Continue down your body until
you have repeated this with every muscle group.

☐ **Use creative visualization.**
Close your eyes and visualize a pleasant place or
experience and put yourself there. Imagine what it
sounds like, smells like, feels like, and looks like in your
mind's eye.

☐ **Practice gentle movement.**
Engage in an activity that lets you move and relaxes
you at the same time, like yoga, tai chi, or a silent walk.
Many times it is easier for an adrenaline junkie to relax
by channeling their energy into some kind of physical
activity instead of sitting still.

[Your Care Plan]

1 Are you stressed? Circle all of the stress exhaustion symptoms
listed in the table chart on page 94 that you have experienced

consistently in the last thirty days. Does anything surprise you? Are you any more stressed than you were aware of previously?

Physical	Spiritual	Emotional/ Cultural	Creative
Aerobic exercise	Children	Ceremony	Craft
Horseback riding	Church	Concerts	Drawing/ singing/dancing
Fishing	Chanting/ Meditation	Drumming	
Martial arts		Movies	Keeping a journal
Massage	Nature	Museums	
Rock climbing	Pets	Music	Knitting, crocheting
Weight training	Rituals	Playing games	Painting
Yoga, tai chi, qi gong		Reading	Playing a musical instrument
		Theatre	Pottery
			Woodworking

2 Practice the relaxation exercises described earlier: Conscious breathing, progressive relaxation, creative visualization, or gentle movement. Decide which one works best for you and consciously practice it wherever you can—in your office, at home, in traffic, even in the dentist's chair.

3 Many other activities, exercises, and interests can help you with your relaxation. Look at the table below and circle what appeals to you when you need a diversion, distraction, or relaxation opportunity.

4 Think about someone you know who is laid-back and the true antithesis of an adrenaline junkie. This is someone you respect for their "quiet energy." They are very effective in what

they do, but not with the same frenzy and chaos familiar to an adrenaline junkie. Talk with them; ask them what their days are like and how they act and react.

What does having quiet energy look like for you? How could you choose to live with less chaos, crisis, and stress in your life? Practice your own quiet energy for a full day and write about how it feels.

Chapter 9

Inserting a Pacemaker

"Where you are headed is more important
than how fast you are going..."
—Stephen R. Covey

Pacing ourselves is differentiating between being able to do *any-thing* and trying to do *everything*. We are capable of doing anything (well, almost) we set our minds to, but we can't do everything. It is humanly impossible, and when we try to do everything, we end up living life like an emergency.

Pacing yourself doesn't require you to give up the things you love; in fact, it is just the opposite. Pacing affords you enough time and energy for the things that give you the most joy and fulfillment, the things that matter most. As my dear friend and coach, Belle, says so well, "You can have it all, you just have to pick your all." Effective pacing allows you to pick your all.

Pacing ourselves relates to how fast or slow we live, and what and how much we put into our lives. It requires a deli-cate balance, because not having enough going on can be just as stressful as having too much. Writing this book forced me to reexamine my own pacing. Even though I purposely cleared my calendar of many activities to permit more time for my writing, I still needed some social contact or I felt lonely and disconnected.

When we don't pace ourselves, we try to do everything by cramming too many things into one day, doing more than one thing at a time, and trying to do everything faster. We end up flitting from one activity to the next, and get frustrated, disappointed, and burned out in the process.

Effective Pacing

When we pace ourselves effectively, we follow the natural ebb and flow of life and maintain different energy levels for different requirements. We acknowledge the full spectrum of life's activities by accommodating the fast and busy periods as well as appreciating the slower and quieter ones. Different circumstances and stages of our lives will require that we adjust our pacing to accommodate change.

> Marge had lived in Colorado most of her adult life. She loved the abundance of year-round outdoor physical activity and she passionately participated in outdoor sports and events. Marge led a busy and active life, traveling weekly for her job and spending her weekends in the mountains on the bike path, hiking trails, or the ski slopes.
>
> When Marge was transferred to the Midwest and experienced her first harsh winter, her life changed radically. She traveled much less and had far fewer opportunities for outdoor activity. She had to let go of her familiar fast and active pace of living. She told me, "This was an opportunity for me to slow down and focus on some areas in my life I never took the time for before. I have a beautiful garden, a stable relationship, and love being at home, now more than ever."

Marge left a very active and busy life in Colorado and traded it in for a more quiet and slower life in Indiana. Both lives are full, in their own right, but each one has its own unique pace. By effectively pacing herself in her new environment, Marge could appreciate slowing down and saw it as an opportunity to focus on and experience new and exciting aspects of herself and her life.

Keeping Pace

When a patient's heartbeat becomes erratic and beats either too fast or too slow, an electronic pacemaker is used to help regulate the heartbeat and return it to a normal, healthy rhythm. These pacemakers can be internal or external. Internal pacemakers are permanent and are surgically placed under the skin. External pacemakers serve as temporary solutions and are worn outside of the body.

We pace ourselves internally and externally, too. Internal pacing comes from within us, when we initiate and follow through according to our own internal rhythms. External pacing comes from outside influences, from the people and situations in our lives. We have to take control over internally and externally pacing ourselves.

Internal Rhythms: Internal Pacing

We take full responsibility for internally pacing ourselves by honoring our internal rhythms. This includes paying attention to when our physical energy level peaks, when it plummets, and when it levels out. We can correlate our energy levels with our sleep patterns, social calendar, or work schedule to stay in tune with our internal rhythms. When we become aware of our internal rhythm, we can schedule our most demanding activities during our highest energy levels. My energy level is highest in the morning, and I would never think of working out or doing a lot of writing in the evening, when I am winding down and thinking about bedtime!

Internally pacing ourselves also requires us to pay attention to our emotional capacity and limitations. This is recognizing when you need to take a break, a rest, a recovery period to rejuvenate yourself, and then taking it. Just like an electronic pacemaker, we are ineffective if we don't recharge our batteries. We just don't have anything to give when our batteries are dead!

To be effective at internally pacing ourselves, we have to look at the big picture, the big plan. When you schedule activities, don't just refer to the week. Look at the whole month, or even an entire season (especially during the holidays) before you commit yourself. I have a monthly and yearly calendar I consult with before I add anything to my schedule.

Pacing yourself effectively also gives you the freedom to change your mind. Most of us take our commitments seriously and never want to let anyone down, but there are times when you need to change your mind. If you are feeling pressed and stressed about a commitment, strongly consider rescheduling or canceling it to honor your own internal pacing. You may find it provides a welcome relief to everyone involved.

Internally pacing yourself is critical in mountain climbing. I learned to really appreciate the importance of pacing after not doing it myself.

Keeping with my competitive spirit, I always used to try to keep up with the leaders of the pack on a climb, by pushing myself and ignoring my physical discomforts. I struggled to get to the top.

On one particularly difficult climb, I started out like I always did, full of anticipation, excitement, and energy. But the higher we climbed, the steeper the grade, the thicker the air, and the more fatigued I felt.

I hadn't paced myself with my food, water, or rest, so I "bonked." For climbers, "bonking" is feeling totally exhausted; dizziness, headache, and nausea are common. All I could think about was getting down. I made it to the top, but I felt really lousy.

On my next climb, I consciously paced myself, taking rest when I needed it and staying fueled with food and water. I eased my way to the top, feeling great the whole time. I realized that pacing is critical to the whole mountain-climbing experience.

Internal pacing is also critical to our whole life experience. We can ease our way to the top, and enjoy the climb without so much struggling if we learn how to internally pace ourselves effectively.

Outside Influences: External Pacing

Externally pacing ourselves involves all of the outside influences in our lives, including our relationships, our life situations, and the expectations everyone else has of us. Even with our most prudent internal pacing, we may need a little help from our friends. The people in our lives can pace us externally by setting an example for us, or mirroring our behavior back to us when we don't see it. My husband and I have vastly different internal rhythms, but he can sense when I am not pacing myself effectively, and will remark on it, gently reminding me to make the appropriate adjustments.

Surrounding yourself with other successful pacers can help you with your own external pacing. Many people are proficient at pacing their own lives and you can learn a lot from them by observing their pacing skills and deciding which ones you want to adopt. You might even ask them to be your gatekeeper during a particularly stressful time, to keep you accountable for your own pacing.

Outside influences can also hinder our effective pacing. Overbearing bosses, needy neighbors, and people who demand more from us than we can give, or pace us too fast, threaten our internal rhythms. In these circumstances, we have to override these external forces and rely solely on our internal rhythms.

We also need to override someone else's pace if it is not comfortable for us. This means setting your boundaries with your pace. If someone is pushing you too hard and fast, or dragging you down by going painfully slow, let them know it. There are people I choose not to climb with because they cannot keep a pace that is comfortable for me.

Beware of people who can't pace their own lives! You know the type—the ones who try to do everything, and end up frustrated, disappointed, and burned out. They can have a negative influence on you and they are not the kind of people you want to surround yourself with to externally pace your life effectively.

[Your Care Plan]

1 What comes up for you when you think about pacing? List at least ten words that pop into your head. Is pacing a positive goal to aspire to, or does it feel negative—too hard or too slow? Pay close attention to your own judgments about pacing as you do the following exercises.

2 How are you pacing yourself internally? Keep an energy log for one week. Include the time you get up, your energy levels throughout the day, and the time you go to bed. This is how you can correlate your energy levels with your sleep patterns, your social calendar, and your work schedule. Evaluate your pacing: It is too fast, too slow, or just right?

Example:

Date	Waking Time	Hours slept	Mid-morning	Mid-afternoon	Bedtime	Pacing
Monday, January 7	5:30 a.m. tired, hit snooze x 3	6	Moderate	Low	9:00 p.m.	exhausted Too fast
Tuesday, January 8	7:00 a.m. rested, no alarm	8	High	High	10:00 p.m.	Good, just right

Energy Log

Date	Waking Time	Hours slept	Mid-morning	Mid-afternoon	Bedtime	Pacing

3 How are you pacing yourself externally?

Do you have external pacers who help you with your comfortable pace?

Have you let them know what a support they are to you?

If you don't already have an external pacer, think of a successful pacer in your life. Ask them how they pace their lives. Ask if she would be your gatekeeper to help you externally pace yourself.

Are there any external pacemakers pacing you too slow or too fast right now? Tell them what you need from them if you feel you are being pushed ahead or held back at a pace that does not allow you to honor your internal rhythms.

Chapter 10

The Disaster Plan

"Any idiot can face a crisis. It's this
day-to-day living that wears you out."
—Anton Chekhov

*E*very ER has a disaster plan to handle special circumstances that would overtax the normal systems they have in place. This plan includes notifying the trauma team for additional support personnel, having back-up supplies readily available, and coordinating the whole effort to provide an efficient and organized operation.

We cannot handle a disaster in our everyday life by ourselves any more than we can handle a disaster alone in the ER. An illness, accident, loss—anything that stresses our normal systems—can be classified as a disaster. When you have the flu and can't lift your head off the bed, your kids still have to go to school and soccer practice. When your car is totaled, you still have to find a way to buy groceries. When a loved one dies, you need to process your grief, anger, and guilt with someone. All of these situations stress the normal systems we have in place and require us to get support. When we have our own personal disaster plan in place, we are prepared to get the support we need.

Our personal disaster plan must be solid enough to handle any situation that overwhelms us and prevents us from getting our needs met. The word "disaster" brings to mind catastrophic and devastating circumstances, but the plan is in place to head off additional catastrophe and allow us to be proactive in our approach. The ER disaster plan is developed for all different kinds of situations, from a massive school shooting to a summer camp plagued with food poisoning.

> The call came in the middle of the ER night shift from a camp nurse who was overwhelmed with twenty-two teenage campers experiencing severe gastrointestinal symptoms. They all complained of abdominal cramping, nausea and vomiting, and diarrhea, approximately six hours after eating their last meal. These are all classic symptoms for food poisoning.
>
> Since everyone had eaten the same thing, and the camp enrolled a total of 120 campers plus another thirty-five staff members, the ER disaster plan was activated in preparation for treating a potentially large number of patients with food poisoning.

Hospitals are very liberal in activating their disaster plans and it isn't necessary for us to wait for things to escalate in our everyday lives to activate our own personal disaster plan. It's always better to have back-up resources and not need them than to really need them and not have them. The whole idea of creating our personal disaster plan is to be proactive in our preparation and support.

Creating Your Personal Disaster Plan

Just like the ER, you must have your personal disaster plan in place before a disaster strikes. It is impossible to make decisions and follow rational processes when you're caught in the middle of a crisis without a plan. Disaster plans are well thought out and reasonably written in preparation for the worst. Creating your disaster plan means organizing your trauma team to get additional support, stocking your crash cart to have back-up supplies readily available, and coordinating the whole effort by identifying your "divert" activities. Taking these steps will ensure efficient and organized management of your personal disaster.

Organize Your Trauma Team

The ER trauma team is a group of health care professionals who respond to disasters and includes surgeons, specialty physicians, nurses, respiratory therapists, paramedics, and laboratory and X-ray technicians. In organizing your trauma team, seek out people who can provide you with support, advice, and comfort. Look to your friends, family members, and even mental health professionals whom you can trust unconditionally and rely on in times of need.

When we don't have a trauma team, we're out there all alone. We are more vulnerable to losing our perspective and our capacity to deal with our circumstances. It's not about being weak or not having the ability to tough it out. The fact is, there is strength in numbers. Having someone else to listen to you, to advise and assist you when your normal systems are stressed, is crucial to your disaster plan.

Your trauma team must be made up of people you trust and feel comfortable asking for help. It's not always easy for us to ask for help when we need it. But it's important to remember that the people who care about us want to help, they just don't always know what to do. Sometimes we can help them help us.

> Two weeks before Christmas, my best friend Martha called to tell me her mother had just passed away. The whole family had been planning to be with her for one last Christmas celebration and now that would not be possible.
>
> Her mother's pain and suffering were over, but what I heard in Martha's voice was her pain just beginning. The funeral was set for the following weekend in Kansas City. After I hung up the phone I thought, "What could I say? What could I send? What could I do that could possibly be a comfort to my best friend in this difficult time?"
>
> I quickly made the decision to fly to Kansas City for the funeral. I called Martha back, fully expecting her to try to talk me out of coming because of the holiday and the expense, but all she said was, "You can't imagine how much that means to me."
>
> I didn't perform any extraordinary duties that weekend since her church congregation provided meals and coordinated the funeral service. My only responsibility was to be my best friend's emotional support.

I felt honored to be able to share my friend's grief and sorrow so intimately with her. It helped me appreciate how much strength and support a trauma team can be in our lives.

You can ask your spouse and immediate family for help, but don't expect one person to fulfill all your needs. Consider the rich variety of resources you have available to you for your trauma team—family, friends, lovers, colleagues and coworkers, spiritual leaders, counselors, and medical professionals. This is a team effort, and you need a variety of resources to call on. Invite them to be part of your personal disaster plan; chances are, they'll be happy to help you, and honored to be asked.

Stock Your Crash Cart

The ER crash cart consists of medications, supplies, and all the equipment necessary for a resuscitation. It would never work to have to hunt down and gather the necessary supplies during a disaster. Just like the ER, we need to have our own back-up provisions readily available in preparation for a disaster.

Your crash cart must have a physical location, but it can be anything from a small box to an entire room. You can stock a special basket with provisions, or create a private, sacred space. Find a room or portion of a room to create a space that invites you to be calm, comfortable, and safe. Surround yourself with your favorite pillows, afghans, candles, aromatherapy, images— anything that gives you comfort and makes you feel good. If you don't have a particular space available to you, take your special box of provisions with you to a church sanctuary, a park, a beach—even a retreat center.

Here are some additional supplies for your crash cart:

- List of your trauma team members with phone numbers
- Books (inspirational readings and escape novels)
- Relaxation or meditation tapes
- Soothing music

- A journal and a nice pen
- Self-nurture supplies (bubble bath, facial, manicure, pedicure, etc.)
- List of your favorite movies to watch or books to read
- Needlepoint, clay, art supplies—whatever medium you use to engage your creativity
- Feel-good file of letters, poems, quotes, cards, pictures— items that have special meaning for you (This idea comes from my good friend and mentor, Mary LoVerde, author of *Stop Screaming at the Microwave!*)
- Hot flavored teas, hot chocolate

You can utilize any or all parts of your crash cart whenever your normal systems are feeling stressed. You may just need ten minutes of quiet time to yourself in a safe, calm space. You may need to watch your favorite gut-wrenching love story and have a good cry. You may need to call a friend and get a different perspective on the blowup you just had with your teenager. You may not know what you need, but if you have your crash cart prepared, you can be open and see what part(s) of it fill your needs at the moment.

Go on Divert

The ER disaster plan can involve going on divert status. This means the ER will no longer accept ambulance patients, and the hospital will not admit patients unless they are directly related to the disaster. Divert status allows the hospital to accommodate and focus on the potentially high number of casualties from the disaster.

Just like the ER, your personal disaster has to be your priority, so you need to divert your other responsibilities and activities. You can divert them to your trauma team, or choose not to have them done at all. People will say, "just let me know if you need anything." Of course they are sincere, but we don't always know where to begin to tell them what we need, especially when our normal systems are so stressed. If you identify responsibilities you can divert up front, you can more easily let people know what you need from them.

Examples of divert responsibilities:

Shop for groceries

Cook meals

Transport children

Baby-sit children

Feed pets

Walk dog

Contact other family members

Pay bills

Research different options (medical, legal, financial)

Run errands

Arrange substitutes for volunteer work

Notify employer of situation

Provide check-ins

Return phone calls to family and friends

Act as gatekeeper

[Your Care Plan]

Now it's time to create your own Personal Disaster Plan.

1 **Organize your trauma team by identifying the members.**
They can be either long distance or next door, but list a min-
imum of five people and include family, friends, and at least
one mental health professional as a resource. If you haven't
already, ask each of them to be part of your trauma team and
explain what role they would play as part of your team.

	Name	Phone Number
1.		
2.		
3.		
4.		
5.		
6.		
7.		
8.		
9.		
10.		

2 **Stock your crash cart.** Start gathering the provisions for your
crash cart that have heart and meaning for you. Review the list
of suggestions on page 113 and add anything else that makes

you feel good. Be sure to include the list of your trauma team members and their phone numbers. If you have an area available in your home, create a sacred space for yourself.

3 **List your divert activities.** Refer to the examples on page 113. These are all the responsibilities you have and would need someone else to take over in the case of a disaster.

_____

_____

_____

_____

_____

_____

_____

_____

_____

_____

_____

_____

_____

_____

Chapter 11

Universal Precautions

"I try to take one day at a time, but sometimes
several days attack me at once."
—Ashleigh Brilliant

Universal precautions is a hospital standard mandating all personnel treat every body fluid as if it were infectious. Health care personnel are expected to wear gloves, gowns, and masks, when appropriate, to prevent exposure to these potentially infectious body fluids. With the intimate contact ER personnel have with their patients and the population at risk for so many different infectious diseases today, universal precautions protect both the staff and the patient.

Using universal precautions in our everyday lives as safety measures and defensive maneuvers can help us protect our time and energy. They help us guard our schedules *ruthlessly* by treating every request, every meeting, and every commitment as a potential threat. Universal precautions are mandatory in your everyday life when you want to stop living life like an emergency.

The ambulance brought in a sixteen-year-old boy who had shot himself with a .38-caliber pistol. He was bleeding profusely and blood splattered everywhere: on the walls, on various pieces of equipment, and on the ER personnel who assisted in the rescue effort.

It was later determined the patient had hepatitis C, a highly contagious liver disease transmitted through the blood. Because this occurred before universal precautions were strictly enforced, every health care provider who had come in contact with this patient had to be tested for hepatitis C.

This would not be a major concern today because of the standard use of universal precautions in all hospitals. It is easy to see what the impact of not using them could be here, since there is no cure for hepatitis C, a debilitating chronic liver disease, and the worst-case scenario requires a liver transplant.

When we don't use universal precautions in our everyday lives, our time is not our own and we end up doing things and spending time in ways that don't matter most to us. We cannot live our priorities and focus our energy on what really counts if we don't safeguard our schedules from everyone and everything.

Here are some specific steps you can take to use universal precautions life and guard your schedule *ruthlessly*.

Eliminate Your Energy Drainers

Energy drainers are those commitments, responsibilities, and relationships that drain our time and energy. They can be friends, coworkers, committees, or chores we commit to that drain our energy stores dry. These drainers have a cumulative effect on our lives because we typically worry about them before they occur, we suffer through them, and agonize over them afterwards. Using universal precautions in our everyday lives doesn't just mean actively choosing what things to add in, it also means choosing what things to take out. We have to eliminate our drainers.

Even something as simple as a phone call can be a drainer. I'm talking about that person who calls you on the phone and goes on and on and on about herself for seventeen minutes straight, until she finally takes a breath and says, "But enough about me, how do you feel—about me?" Caller ID devices can be a great help in detecting this potential drainer, but at some point you just have to come clean before she even gets started and say, "This is just not a good time for me," and of course it will never be a good time for you, so she can call someone else.

Drainers are unique to each individual, and what is draining for one person can be therapeutic for someone else. I have heard of people who actually find housework relaxing, but I find it very draining. I would (almost) rather go to the dentist. I wholeheartedly agree with Phyllis Diller when she says, "Housework probably won't kill you, but why take the chance?" I am a big believer in getting domestic help. (More on this later.)

Clutter is a drainer. When our outside environment is chaotic, our inside condition is chaotic. When we're surrounded by clutter, we lose the confidence to throw anything away, just in case we might need it someday. If we ever do need it, chances are we won't be able to find it anyway. It's a vicious cycle, and the more clutter we accumulate, the less confident we feel, and the more clutter we accumulate. There are actually professionals you can pay to come into your home and help you get rid of your clutter!

I used to save things, thinking I'd have a garage sale someday, which of course never happened and I continued to accumulate more clutter. Ironically, even having a garage sale can be a huge drainer; you have to gather your stuff together, price it, and then sit there all day, listening to buyers try to bargain you down on the price. I've learned to just call the Salvation Army with the turn of every season; four times a year, they come right to my door, pick up my clutter, and give me a receipt for a tax write-off.

Home improvement projects that you try to do yourself so you can save money are drainers. It always takes far longer and costs much, much more than you expect it to. One of my clients told me her husband had been remodeling the kitchen—for the last two years. She was forced to wash dishes in the tub and cook everything in the microwave for most of that time.

I handle this potential drainer by refusing to allow my husband to do any more home improvement projects after it took him six months to tile our shower stall. It wasn't as bad as doing dishes, but I had to wash my hair in the tub for half a year. We now happily pay professionals to do the job much more efficiently, and sometimes even more cheaply.

Postpone Your Yes

If you have trouble saying no because you feel obligated, guilty, or even because it sounds like something your really want to do, *never* say yes to anything on the spot. Make a habit to postpone your yes by simply saying, "I'll have to get back to you on that."

We often say yes without thinking it through because it's easier—at least in the short term—than saying no. When you say yes to one thing, you are saying no to something else. Postponing your yes gives you the chance to evaluate your schedule and your energy, and decide if you honestly want to participate in what is being asked of you.

When you decide your answer is no, then say, "I'm sorry I won't be able to do that," or "I'm flattered that you asked me, but I have to decline," and leave it at that. You don't need to go into a convoluted explanation about your dying dog or your sick mother-in-law. Keep it simple and appreciate the rewards of saying no.

When I started working in the ER, I was ambitious and energetic, eager to please and get "seasoned" with experience. The charge nurse always called me first whenever they needed extra help, and I would come in early, stay late, and even work on my day off.

After a few months and a lot of overtime, I realized my days off were too few and far between and I was spending them trying to catch up on sleep, laundry, and long-neglected chores. I felt like all I did was work and then recover from work. After a few times of saying no to working extra hours so I could ride my bike or spend time with my friends, the charge nurse stopped calling me.

Give up Your Guilt

Guilt drains us by keeping us stuck in thinking and feeling badly about ourselves. When we feel guilty about all the things we haven't done, we end up "shoulding" on ourselves. It is by choice we take the responsibility of caring for everything and everyone else, and it is by choice that we can let it go.

We often feel guilty when we put our needs first; we think we are "being selfish." Using universal precautions and actively choosing what and who we want in our lives isn't being selfish, it's being true to ourselves. Being true to ourselves gives us the capacity to give more to others without feeling resentment or bitter obligation.

> Alice was well accomplished in the guilt department. She not only took care of all of her family's basic needs, she also felt solely responsible for making sure they always had a good time at family gatherings, holidays, and vacations.
>
> One year Alice realized how much she dreaded their family vacations. Not only did she pack everyone's clothing and plan all of the meals, she also made sure everyone was having fun.
>
> After organizing her family for that year's trip, she made the drastic decision to stay home and take a vacation by herself.
>
> Even though her family came back two days early, Alice received them with open arms. Instead of feeling exhausted and resentful, this vacation left her feeling renewed and refreshed. Alice now spends one family vacation a year at home by herself, without feeling guilty.

Utilize OPT

OPT stands for "other people's time" (and expertise). There is nothing wrong with asking for a little help if you aren't very good at doing something, or you just don't like doing it, which usually are one in the same. For me, this is the housecleaning I alluded to earlier.

Hiring a finishing man, a housecleaner, or whichever expert you need to help you with an activity that drains your time and energy is totally acceptable and encouraged in universal precautions. It is important to remember that time is money, and when you save time (and energy), you save money.

My husband is an engineer, and if you know anything about engineers, you know they believe any project worth doing is worth overdoing. He is methodical, meticulous, thorough, and incredibly slow at everything he does.

I've already mentioned my distaste for housecleaning and after my futile attempts, my husband decided he would take over the responsibility. He did a great job, and because he is so methodical, meticulous, thorough, and incredibly slow, it took him the entire weekend to clean the house. That wouldn't have been so bad, except that he complained about it all weekend.

After a lot of convincing, my husband finally agreed to hire a cleaning lady on a trial basis. We couldn't really afford a cleaning lady, but the way I looked at it, we couldn't afford not to get one. It has been five years, and even though we've been through many cleaning ladies, I am proud to say we still have one.

We utilized OPT so that we can spend our time and energy on the weekend doing the things that matter most.

Create the Space

You are the only one who can take responsibility for being *ruthless* with your schedule. I've discussed how important it is to keep a balance of activities in your life, that when you add something into your life, you have to take something out to allow space for it. Otherwise, the activities you want to take part in won't be as enjoyable because you won't have the time and energy for them.

Sara came to see me because she wanted to "get organized." We started by talking about how she spent her time and energy as she reviewed her daily routine. Sara definitely had a full life, but her schedule didn't seem too unreasonable.

Almost as an afterthought, she mentioned she was getting married in six months. She had dreamed of a big storybook wedding ever since she was a little girl, and she was determined to have one. To complicate matters, it was taking place out of state, in her hometown. But her biggest stressor was handling every detail of the wedding by herself, because her family did not approve of her fiancé.

This significant event in Sara's life mattered most, but she neglected to create any space for it emotionally or physically. We talked about what Sara could give up or postpone until after the wedding. She decided to cancel her dance class, postpone her initiation into a new service club, and hold off pursuing a promotion at her company. Sara thanked me for helping her "get organized."

Bring Back Your Joys

The whole reason we want to utilize universal precautions in our everyday lives is to have time for the things that matter most, the true joys in our lives. We talk about what is most important, what we really love, and what we are passionate about, but how much time and energy are we *really* devoting to it? The only way you can bring back your joys is to take out your drainers, postpone your yes, give up your guilt, utilize OPT, and create the space. Start with any of these and you are on your way to guarding your schedule *ruthlessly!*

[Your Care Plan]

1 Postpone your yes to at least one activity or request this week. Say, "I'll have to get back to you on that," even if you think you really want to do it. Notice whether you feel different about your decision after you have the chance to evaluate the time and energy you have to devote to it. Keep track of how many times you say no when you have an opportunity to fully evaluate the activity.

2 Make a list of the energy drainers in your life right now. Be very specific and include both your professional and personal life. List whatever comes up for you, no matter how insignificant it may seem.

3 Apply universal precautions to the drainers in your life: *What could you say no to?*

What do you need to give up the guilt about?

How could you utilize OPT?

What do you need to let go of to create the space?

Example:

Drainers	Universal Precaution
Clutter in my office	Organize office with friend or professional organizer
Negative coworker	Set limits and boundaries
Tooth that is bothering me	Make dentist appointment
Lack of communication	Schedule a specific meeting with my agenda with my boss
60-minute commute to work every day	Listen to inspirational tapes/rehearse speech
Training new puppy	Give up volunteer job at library/Start obedience school
Book club	Take a break for three months, then re-evaluate
House work	Hire a housekeeper
Christmas cards	Choose not to send cards at the holidays
Car making a funny noise	Schedule appointment with mechanic

Drainers	Universal Precaution

4 It is important to identify and remember what matters most to you in your life right now. List the joys in your life, the things you love and have a passion for. After you make your list, write down how much time you actually spend with these joys. Using universal precautions will allow you more time and the energy for what matters most.

Example:

Joys in my Life	Hours each week/month/year
My husband	10 hours/week
My nephews	1 week/year
My dog	10 hours/week
Reading	5 hours/week
Best friends	3 hours/week
Exercise	6 hours/week
Women's Retreat	2 weekends/year
Cooking	5 hours/week
Football	3 hours/week
Yoga	3 hours/week

Joys in my Life	Hours each week/month/year

Joys in my Life	Hours each week/month/year

Chapter 12

Take a Break

"We withdraw, not only from the concerns
of the world and its preoccupations but from the
incessant monologue and concerns within ourselves,
in order for something else to come into being."

—Deena Metzger

The emotional needs of patients and their families can sometimes be the most demanding part of working in the ER.
Because of the nature of circumstances that bring people to the
ER, staff frequently share the most intimate and private moments with them. There is a huge responsibility in providing
both the emotional support and the medical care for these patients and it takes its toll.

A nineteen-year-old girl was brought in by ambulance after a
head-on collision. Running late for work, she lost control of
her car while trying to pass a truck.

There wasn't a visible scratch on her, but she suffered massive internal injuries too extensive to survive. After it was ev-
ident she could not be successfully resuscitated, the most
difficult part of the effort remained: telling her parents, who
anxiously waited in the chapel.

The kind of emotional intensity involved in telling the parents of a nineteen-year-old girl that their daughter could not be

saved necessitates getting away from the immediate environment and taking a break. There were plenty of shifts when I toughed it out and "made it" without a break. But when I did manage to get away, I always came back refreshed and revived, and had more to give to everyone else. I became very conscientious about taking my breaks and relieving other staff members for theirs.

We need to take a break in our everyday lives too, and the busier we are and the less time we think we have to take one, the more likely we need it. A break provides us with a pause, a breather, and even a vacation away from our everyday lives to have the opportunity to reflect, renew, and recover.

When we don't take breaks, we can easily lose our perspective and become resentful and bitter. We can also lose our edge, our focus, and our ability to perform well. We all need mental, emotional, and physical rest to recharge ourselves, and a break can provide this.

Many times when we are feeling tired and low on energy, we think we just need more sleep. Instead of being physically worn out, we may be emotionally or mentally exhausted, or both. Sleep alone will not necessarily take care of mental and emotional fatigue. We need to take a break from our everyday routines, responsibilities, and requirements to restore ourselves mentally and emotionally.

Taking a break in our everyday lives can include stopping for as little as five minutes (see Chapter 3), creating an intentional afternoon (see Chapter 6), or going on a weekend retreat. They all serve a distinct purpose, and all are valuable. Taking a break is difficult for many of us, so I suggest you start out small, and build from there. If you can't find five minutes in your day to stop, it is totally unreasonable to ask you to plan a weekend retreat!

Here are some different ways we can take breaks in our lives.

Take Five

Many years ago, when I was a smoker, I would never have missed that cigarette break, but when I quit smoking, instead of substituting a five-minute breather for a smoke, I skipped it altogether. I really missed it and resented the other smokers who made sure they got theirs. Taking just five minutes to get away from your immediate environment is very rejuvenating.

You can physically leave your work area by taking a walk around the office, going outside to breathe in fresh air, or going to another room, floor, or building to rest and be quiet. You can take a mental break by staying where you are and stopping for five minutes to check in with yourself, as long as you're sure no one will interrupt you. Focus on your breathing and take a mental vacation from whatever you are doing. Even this quick five-minute break can give you a new perspective and sense of restoration.

Take Lunch

It always amazes to me to learn how many people don't take lunch. I don't consider it "taking lunch" if you're answering the phone, writing a memo, and preparing for a meeting while you wolf down a sandwich. Taking lunch is getting away from your immediate work area, away from the phone, away from your "in" and "out" boxes and countless other distractions. If you don't leave your area for a break at lunch, you're just not taking lunch. Just walking down the hall a few feet away from your immediate area to eat your sandwich is a break. Getting outside to breathe some fresh air and even taking a little walk is better still.

If you don't think you have time to take lunch, bear this in mind: Productivity studies have shown how much more we accomplish when we stay fresh and alert. We can do this by keeping ourselves fueled with food and water, and taking breaks.

Take an Afternoon

This is half-day of respite and can be a morning or afternoon, although it is nice to get whatever you need to get done in the morning, and feel more at ease in the afternoon. You can choose to stay home in your sacred space (see Chapter 10), or venture out to somewhere restful, safe and comforting.

If you choose to stay at home, be firm about this being your break and not an opportunity to make phone calls, do chores, or catch up on bills. This is time for you to relax, rest, and restore, not to focus on getting things done. Curl up and read, do artwork, write, play a musical instrument, spend time in the garden—do whatever you like, as long as these activities help you relax and don't feel like work to you.

Take a Day

A whole day? Yes, a whole day. Taking a break for a full day allows you some time to transition into your break time, and allows your mind and body to slow down. This is a whole day for you to create an intentional experience (see Chapter 6) for yourself to do exactly as you please.

You will decide what your day looks like for you. Just like the half-day, you can choose to stay home, or make plans to get away. If you travel a lot, home will feel like a respite, as long as you don't turn it into a catch-up day. If you need to get out of the house, choose somewhere that speaks to you, in nature, a museum or even a retreat center for the day. Go or be wherever you can feel like you are honestly taking a break for the whole day.

Take a Retreat

The absolute ultimate break we can give ourselves is a weekend retreat. Retreats offer an opportunity to get away and seek refuge from the distractions, interruptions, and responsibilities tugging at you at home. You can go somewhere that speaks to you, feels safe, and feeds your soul. The mountains are my favorite place to retreat, but the beach, the desert, or a cabin in the woods can offer the same peace and solitude.

We can retreat by ourselves or in an organized group. If you retreat with a group, it is essential that you have the privacy and freedom to do exactly what you want, even if you don't know what that is before you go. Too much structure and activity won't allow you to focus fully on yourself and attend to your needs.

The first retreat I ever participated in was more like a boot camp. I had a great time, I just didn't have a retreat. We started every day at sunrise with power yoga, then on to the pool for laps. After lunch, we went single-track mountain-biking, followed by a challenging trail run.

I have never pushed myself so hard physically or ate such large quantities of food in my life. I thought I was in fairly good shape at the time, but I knew I was in trouble when a large group gathered for a ten-mile run after our first rigorous day of retreat.

I came home exhausted and sore, instead of refreshed and renewed. I realized my life and my exercise program are intense enough without needing to add a week-long training camp. What I really needed was a retreat, and now I know where to go to get it.

Different retreat settings offer us different experiences. I go to a yoga center and sleep in a dormitory when I want to deepen my yoga and meditation practice in a more structured, communal environment. I go to a guest ranch and stay in a cabin by myself when I want to create my own schedule and have more solitude. Each place is unique, but both offer quiet, safe and clean accommodations with delicious meals.

Women's Mountain Retreats

I never fully appreciated how powerful a retreat can be until I started facilitating my own Women's Mountain Retreats. Seeing the transformation that takes place in these women within just a couple of days compels me to have the next one. After making extensive arrangements and preparations to get themselves there, most of the women arrive that Friday evening exhausted and tentative, not knowing quite what to expect from the weekend. But by the end of that first evening, they are transformed into relaxed and open beings, and intuitively understand why they are there.

The Women's Mountain Retreats I facilitate give women the opportunity to get away to the mountains and focus totally on themselves for a full weekend. They all get a private room and three homemade meals a day, and enjoy activities like horseback riding, hiking, massage, yoga, and sharing circles. All the activities are optional, and the women are encouraged to participate as much or as little as they choose.

When I talk about my retreats to anyone the common response I get is, "Oh, that sounds like *exactly* what I need, but I don't have that kind of money…" or "…but I don't have the time," or any of the other *buts* that get in the way. Once the women get there, though, they realize the value of their investment almost immediately. Whether it is for rest, quiet time, or connection, the women consistently tell me they get exactly what they need.

Give Yourself Permission

The hardest part of taking a retreat is giving yourself the permission to go. We seem to have a hard time spending the time and money on ourselves for what seems like such a frivolous and indulgent endeavor. We need to accept that retreating is essential to our well-being and enriches our lives, both personally and professionally. And we're not the only ones to benefit from taking a retreat; the rejuvenation and energy we bring back from the retreat can affect those close to us.

Jill came to see me for help with some health issues complicated by her fibromyalgia, an autoimmune disease that causes severe fatigue and chronic pain. I was planning my very first Women's Mountain Retreat and Jill really wanted to come. She went home to tell her husband all about it, but he wasn't exactly warm and fuzzy about the idea.

Jill knew this retreat was something she really needed, and she didn't give up on going. For the first time since she could remember, she focused on taking care of herself for an entire weekend. She didn't participate in a lot of the group activities and instead chose to nap, read, and enjoy lots of quiet time. The weekend gave her a chance to rest physically and renew herself emotionally and spiritually.

Since that first year, Jill has been back to every one of my retreats. Now her husband encourages her to go every year by writing the check. He realizes not only how much Jill benefits from it, but how much more she has to give to him and the rest of the family after she takes a break.

We often don't realize how much we need to get away, until we get away. You can't wait for the perfect time to schedule a retreat, because there isn't one. There will always be a reason not to go, so schedule the date and work the rest of your life around your retreat date. Honor your commitment to yourself and don't cancel or postpone taking the retreat unless truly dire circumstances arise.

When I was very close to finishing this book, I told a good friend how stressed I was and how I couldn't wait to take myself on a retreat after my book was complete. "Why are you waiting to go?" she asked. "Maybe you really need to take a break now, before you can finish your book."

There is nothing like having your own advice recited back to you, especially when it's right on. I did go on a retreat before I finished this book, and came home refreshed and renewed enough to turn in my manuscript ahead of schedule.

No matter what kind of a break you choose to take—a half-hour, a half-day, or a whole weekend—there are certain supplies and provisions you can take with you. It is important to think about getting your needs met, to nurture yourself physically, mentally, emotionally, and spiritually during your break

What do I need for my break?

──────────────── **[R**x**]** ────────────────

- ☐ Favorite snacks. Take crunchy foods like apples and carrots as well as comfort foods like puddings and soups. (I'm always surprised how hungry I find myself on retreat.)
- ☐ Water, juices, hot teas, hot cocoa.
- ☐ A plan for your meals. Prepare something ahead of time, order out, eat at the Retreat Center, or a plan to cook very simply.
- ☐ A journal (and a nice pen) for writing, drawing, or doodling.
- ☐ Assortment of books or magazines (non–work-related), ranging in thought and intellect. Different readings attract you at different times during your retreat.
- ☐ Something creative you enjoy doing: colored pencils, paints, glitter, magazines (for collages), needlepoint, clay, etc.
- ☐ Aromatic candles.

- Favorite music.

- Favorite lotions and potions to give yourself a facial, pedicure, or long hot bath.

- Walking shoes or boots. Moving your body will open you up physically and emotionally.

- Comfortable, loose clothing you can layer for wearing indoors and outdoors.

- An appointment for a massage or other special treatment.

- Resist bringing cell phones and pagers, and engaging in e-mail correspondence if at all possible.

[Your Care Plan]

These exercises can be done with an afternoon, a whole day, or a weekend break. I highly recommend they be a part of your break, as they will help you process and experience your time in a more meaningful way.

Before Your Break

1 Practice taking a break by taking five minutes during the day, and then taking a lunch. Then look at your calendar and schedule a more extensive break for yourself. If a weekend seems too overwhelming, then start with a half-day or a full day. You will soon discover why I highly recommend a weekend, as it does take a period of transition to get into your break. Stick to your plan for your break and trust that the time you go will be perfect.

2 Set your intention for your break (see Chapter 6). As you
   begin your break, finish the following statements to help you
   set your intention. Be aware that your intention is not written
   in stone and can change during your break; your intention
   may become more apparent to you as time goes on. You may
   have totally different responses when you go back to these
   same questions a day, or even an hour later.

   I am taking this break because...
   Example: ...I need some time to myself.

   _____

   I am most anxious or worried about...
   ...feeling bored or lonely.

   _____

   I am really excited about...
   ...having the time to write in my journal.

   _____

   What I feel I really need from this break is
   ...rest and quiet time.

   _____

   To be present for this break I need to let go of...
   ...feeling guilty about leaving my family.

   _____

During Your Break

3 Notice how you are feeling during your break. It takes a while
   to transition into a slower and quieter existence than what
   you may be used to, so be gentle with yourself. It is perfectly
   normal to have feelings of fatigue, hunger, or loneliness
   during your break.

   Welcome this opportunity to focus on yourself and feel
   what is going on without the usual responsibilities and distractions of your life. Before your break is over and you return to your normal schedule and routine, write about what
   had true heart and meaning for you.

I am feeling...
Example: ...really tired and hungry.

_____

I am learning
...how to be with myself.

_____

This break helped me
...understand where I am in my life.

_____

This break was special for me because
...I was able to do exactly what I wanted to do.

_____

My next break will be different because

...*I will take one more day.*

My next break will be the same with

...*the location. It was perfect.*

After Your Break

4 Think about what part of your break you would like to take back to your everyday life. What could you bring home and incorporate into your daily routine? What had such a powerful influence, you are willing to give something else up to do it?

Examples:

Practice yoga every morning

Write daily in my journal

Take a long, hot bath at least once a week

Get a massage at least once a month

Get more sleep

Drink more water

Take a walk in silence once a week

Practice my stopping exercise five minutes a day

5 Upon returning home, gently ease back into your everyday life instead of jumping right into your normal responsibilities and routines. Don't rush home to cook a meal or unpack and do laundry. Order dinner out and take the time to share your

experiences with your friends or family. This will help them feel involved and help you continue to process the experiences of your break.

6 While you are still feeling the positive effects of your break, schedule the next one. A quarterly break of a day or more is optimal, but twice a year is a reasonable goal.

Chapter 13

The Pain Scale

"My pain has prodded me along my journey."

—Maureen Brady

We use a pain scale in the ER for patients to rate their own discomfort because pain is so subjective. What one person rates as mild pain, another will rate as the most excruciating pain imaginable. Many factors contribute to a person's pain threshold, including their anxiety level, cultural background, and medical history.

The pain scale provides an important diagnostic tool in the ER. Decisions for tests, medications, and even surgery are based on the level of pain rated by the patient. This is particularly true for burn patients, whose prognosis improves with the more pain they experience, since the most severe burn, called a third-degree burn, affects all layers of skin including the nerve endings, and prevents the patient from feeling any pain.

An obviously distraught older man brought in his eight-year-old grandson, who had just "jumped off a cliff." We later learned it was actually a big rock the boy fell from and he landed on both of his hands instead of his feet. His left hand was dangling from his wrist and his right wrist was grossly swollen. I asked him to rate his pain on a scale of one to ten, and he quietly replied, "One or two."

Amazingly calm and collected, the boy refused any pain medication and tried to console his anxious grandfather. X-rays confirmed both wrists were broken severely enough to require surgery. This brave little boy started to cry only when he found out he couldn't eat lunch before he went to surgery.

Later the same day, a middle-aged man rushed into the triage area holding his hands up in the air to protect them from touching anything. "I have to get something for this pain immediately!" he wailed. When I asked him to show me his hands, I braced myself for something horrendous. What I saw were several thorns embedded in the palms of his hands. He had been pulling weeds without wearing gloves and came across a thorn bush. When I asked him to rate his pain on a scale of one to ten, he replied, "Pretty close to ten."

Facing Your Emotional Pain

Each of us has pain in our everyday lives. We hurt physically and we hurt emotionally—from our losses, disappointments, betrayals, or failures. This chapter is about emotional pain, because it can be a lot less obvious and more debilitating to our everyday lives.

Just like physical pain in the ER, emotional pain is highly subjective. People have very different reactions to and display an array of coping mechanisms for emotional pain. I have seen a woman lose her husband of fifty years to a freak auto accident display total acceptance and I have seen a teenager attempt suicide because his girlfriend of two weeks broke up with him.

Emotional pain cannot be quantified. Cultural norms, mental stability, family history, and the individual's learned coping mechanisms are just some of the factors that influence emotional pain tolerance. We don't often think of using a pain scale when it comes to emotional pain, but it can be very useful.

When our emotional pain becomes excruciating (at level 9 or 10), our souls start screaming. This is not an irritating little voice inside our heads (level 1 or 2) we can choose to ignore even if we wanted to. It is our soul crying out for something it desperately needs and is not getting. When our soul screams intensely and loudly enough, we are forced to face our pain, one way or another.

Just like the burn patient whose prognosis is better when they feel a lot of pain, sometimes the more emotional pain we feel, the better it is. Facing our emotional pain is a catalyst for change and helps us to move out of places and situations we no longer need to be in. We are motivated to change unhealthy relationships, dead-end jobs, and destructive behavior patterns when the pain to stay the same becomes too great.

In my early twenties I had been married less than three months when everything changed. My husband quit his day job and started working nights. We received large credit card bills for purchases I had no knowledge of, and got strange phone calls at all hours of the night.

I soon discovered that my husband's erratic behavior was due to his substance abuse. He was heavy into his addiction, and alienating me ensured his using without interruption. My soul was screaming. How could I have made such a terrible mistake?

Ultimately, the pain of staying in that relationship became greater than the pain of leaving it. The sleepless nights and endless arguments forced me to make a decision. When I ended my marriage, I was at the most disappointing and painful point of my life.

The Agonizing Gift

I now realize the experience of my first marriage was an agonizing gift. My pain provided me with a critical turning point. I got counseling, changed jobs, and moved to a different area of the country far better suited to me and my lifestyle.

The agonizing gifts that come with our emotional pain are invaluable. We may not recognize them as gifts while our souls are screaming out in pain, but they can be appreciated later. When you face your emotional pain, you come out on the other side with the lesson, direction, path, or decisions clarified for you.

Another agonizing gift emotional pain gives you is great contrast for the rest of your life. You experience firsthand how you *don't* want to live and how you *don't* want to feel. Just as it is hard to appreciate your health when you're feeling great, it is difficult to appreciate emotional well-being if you don't have anything to compare it to. When you trust that your difficult and intense feelings of pain will pass, you not only appreciate the passing, you also appreciate the agonizing gift.

Emotional pain does not always involve soul screaming. It can come in the form of mild depression, anger, or resentment. When our pain is more subtle, we are at a higher risk because we get used to feeling that way and don't always acknowledge it.

Many times we practice crooked coping mechanisms (see Chapter 7) to avoid our emotional pain. Overeating, overspending, drinking too much, or overdoing any aspect of our lives provides distraction, but only masks our pain. The pain is still there, and the crooked coping mechanisms we adopt only prolong our torment and cause us additional problems.

Confronting Your Pain

We may not be aware of our own emotional pain if it has been with us for a long time or if we subconsciously choose not to face it. It is difficult to remain objective because when we are in pain, whether it is a broken heart or a toothache, we can never imagine being without it and feeling good again. When the pain is gone, we tend to forget how difficult it was and can't imagine feeling that bad again.

Confronting our emotional pain can be a difficult and hurtful process in itself. Having self-acceptance and compassion for our pain instead of self-loathing and resentment frees us to move through the pain and start the healing process. Denying our pain only keeps us stuck in it. We confront our pain by being open to feeling it and honestly answering the difficult questions about it.

When we feel our pain in one area, we feel it in many areas of our lives. When I felt the pain of the failure of my marriage, I grieved for all of the failures in my life, such as not making high school cheerleader or not applying to medical school. Before I could confront my pain, I had to forgive myself for all of my mistakes and perceived failures.

How can I confront my pain?

[R$_x$]

Confronting your pain requires you to dig deep inside yourself and carefully examine what is going on in your head and in your heart. Be gentle with yourself and realize it will take some time. Get quiet and still and ask yourself the following questions:

- What do I need to forgive myself for?
- What mistakes have I made?
- What shame or blame am I carrying?
- Is my soul screaming?
- Do I have a low-grade pain with symptoms of depression, boredom, or loneliness?
- Am I denying myself something?
- Where is my pain?

Answer the above questions by:

- Visualizing your pain as it comes up for you by color, shape, or sound.
- Writing about your pain in stories, poetry, or lists of your feelings.
- Expressing your pain through drawing, painting, doodling, or some other creative outlet.

Healing Your Pain

After we confront our pain, we can start to heal. Many times we need a shift in our perspective to help us heal our pain. We are often too close to it and need a fresh way of looking at it.

Let It Go

You can hang on to your bitterness, resentment, and pain for a lifetime, or you can choose to let it go and move on. Holding on to your resentments has little or no effect on the person or situation you are targeting, but it does have a negative effect on you and keeps you stuck in the pain.

When my husband has hurt my feelings and I choose to brood about it instead of having a meaningful conversation with him, guess which one of us doesn't get any sleep that night?

Choose Your Way

You cannot always be in control of what happens to you, but you can control how you respond to what happens to you. The way you respond to any situation sets up your reality and experience. There are so many incredibly brave role models who survived atrocities of emotional pain in this world and chose to rise above their circumstances. Victor Frankl, a holocaust survivor, says it very well in his book, *Man's Search for Meaning:*

"Everything can be taken from a man but one thing: the last of the human freedoms—to choose one's attitude in any given set of circumstances, to choose one's own way."

Change Your Scenery

You can be your own worst enemy if you spend too much time ruminating about yourself. Focusing on all that is wrong and negative in your life expands it and only brings you more pain and negativity. Get out of your own head and your own way by changing your scenery.

Getting outside in nature is a great way for me to change my perspective. But you may need to do something a little more drastic. Even though they say "wherever you go, there you are," consider changing jobs, relationships, or neighborhoods to get a new perspective.

Have an Attitude of Gratitude

It's so easy to take the basic things for granted like our health, food, and shelter. It's also easy to take peace of mind for granted when we don't have emotional pain in our lives. We need to give thanks for the simple things in life, like having a good day in addition to celebrating all of our bigger blessings. If you can't be grateful for all you have, then you can never have it all.

Move Your Body

Moving your body by walking, running or dancing will open you up both physically and emotionally and can help you let go of your pain. Yoga, tai chi, or martial arts can also empower you to move through your pain with physical and mental exertion.

Get a Second Opinion

Most people realize these days the importance of getting a second opinion for medical attention, especially if the prescribed treatment is invasive or controversial. Medicine is not an exact science, neither is healing your emotional pain.

Sometimes we don't realize our emotional pain because our own symptoms may not be obvious to us. It is often helpful to get a second opinion about your situation from someone you trust. You can choose a close friend or seek professional counseling to help you process your emotional pain.

[Your Care Plan]

We can only treat our pain when we develop an awareness and understanding of it. Because it is on a continuum from intense to lingering and everything in between, the pain scale is a valuable tool to help us evaluate the emotional pain in our everyday lives.

1 Rate the intensity of your emotional pain in the areas listed on a scale of zero to 10, zero being no pain and 10 being the most excruciating pain you can imagine. Specifically identify what comes up for you as you rate each area that you score at 1 or greater. List any crooked coping mechanisms you are using to compensate for your pain.

Example:

Emotion	Rating 0–10	Specifics	Crooked Coping Mechanisms
Loneliness	5	Living in the mountains away from friends/family	Eat too much sugar
Loss	6	Not having children	Blame husband
Not being "enough"	8	Continually challenge myself in my work	Unrealistic expectations

Emotion	Rating 0–10	Specifics	Crooked Coping Mechanisms
Anger			
Anxiety			
Betrayal			
Boredom			
Confusion			
Depression			
Disappointment			
Embarrassment			
Fear			
Feeling worn down			
Grief			
Guilt			
Helplessness			
Hopelessness			
Hurt			
Insecurity			
Loneliness			
Loss			
Mistrust			
Negativity			

Not being enough
_____

Not feeling heard
_____

Not feeling seen
_____

Not feeling understood
_____

Overwhelmed
_____

Regret
_____

Sadness
_____

Self-doubt
_____

Shame
_____

Worry
_____

2 Identify any triggers that bring up your emotional pain.
   Example: The Christmas holidays always trigger my feelings
   of loss over not having children.

   _____

   _____

3 Much of the emotional pain in our lives brings a lesson with
   an agonizing gift. The gift is greater wisdom and a new perspective when we come out on the other side. Identify at least
   one agonizing gift you received from a painful situation, an
   experience, or a circumstance.

   Example: Because I don't have my own children, my ago-
   nizing gift is the special relationship I have developed with my
   nephews. I have a deep appreciation for them when they come

*to Colorado every summer to visit me. We spend a whole
week hiking, biking, backpacking, and playing a ridiculous
amount of putt-putt golf!*

_____

_____

4 Think of five things you are grateful for right now, and write
   them down. Every night before you go to bed, write down
   five different things you are grateful for and do this for seven
   days. Keeping a gratitude journal can give you a different perspective on your emotional pain and on your life in general.

   Today I am grateful for:
   My good health
   My husband's good health
   My relationship with my mom
   My relationship with my nephews
   My opportunity to write and speak about my passion

   _____

   _____

   _____

   _____

   _____

Discharge Instructions

*T*he discharge instructions given to ER patients are a critical component of their treatment plan, and how they are implemented directly affects the outcome. Given both verbally and in written form, they include an explanation of the diagnosis, home care instructions, and any signs and symptoms requiring immediate attention, even a return to the ER.

A forty-year-old cabinetmaker casually wandered in with a bloody towel wrapped around his hand, secured with duct tape. He wasn't wearing protective gloves when he caught his hand in a table saw. When I unwrapped the towel, his fingers looked like ground hamburger.

It took 137 stitches and a lot of imagination for the surgeon to repair his wounds and restore his hand to any level of functioning. His discharge instructions were:

• Keep the dressing clean and dry.

• Look for signs of infection: redness, swelling, pus-filled drainage, or increased pain.

• Return to the ER in 24 hours for a wound check and dressing change.

The initial suturing of the cabinetmaker's hand injury was very successful. But instead of returning to the ER the next day, unfortunately the patient waited two weeks to come back for his wound check and dressing change.

As I peeled the original soiled dressing away, the stench from his wound was almost unbearable. Pus seeped out of the reddened and puffy folds of skin that had been so carefully sewn together two weeks before.

The severe infection he developed required extensive surgery and weeks of intravenous antibiotic therapy. We saved him from an amputation, but after ignoring his discharge instructions, this cabinetmaker's hand was left permanently damaged, with minimal function.

Following through on our own care plans is as critical as following through on the discharge instructions in the ER. This patient did what so many of us do: We seek treatment or advice, get specific instructions on what to do, but then we don't follow through. We take classes and read books to become experts on "how" to do it. We talk about it, write about it, and even counsel others on it, but we skip the most important part: *doing* it. More is *said* than *done*.

By now you've identified all the ways you are living life like an emergency and you realize you need to make some lifestyle changes. You know what to do after reading the rescue strategies presented throughout this book in the prescriptions, the stories, and the care plans. So now what? There is a huge gap between knowing what to do (the information) and following through and doing it (the implementation).

This last chapter provides your discharge instructions for *how* you can overcome your life-threatening lifestyle. How do you get started? How do you stay motivated? How do you deal with your obstacles? How do you know when you are successful, when you are doing it right? Find out by following your discharge instructions which include an assessment of your emergency living, home care instructions on how to follow through, and symptoms requiring your immediate attention.

Emergency Living Assessment

It can be overwhelming trying to figure out what to do with all of the rescue strategies you have learned in this book. Start at the beginning and decide what specific area of your emergency living you want to focus on first. What emergency living behavior, circumstance, or situation is impacting your everyday life the most?

The following statements offer explanations of emergency living correlated with each chapter. The first statement is your subjective assessment and the second statement is the treatment plan you need. Read over them and determine which one speaks to you the loudest. Which sounds the most familiar and the most urgent for you to deal with first? Even though you will only focus on one specific area at a time, prioritize them now so you'll know which order to address them in later.

Assessment: *"I am a rescuer, risk-taker, adrenaline junkie, perfectionist, controller, and driver."*

Treatment: Slow down your life. (See Chapter 1: Emergency Living.)

––––––––––––

Assessment: *"I am a constant procrastinator." "I chronically over-schedule myself."*

Treatment: Make time for the most important things in your life. (See Chapter 2: Triage.)

Assessment: *"I never stop."*

Treatment: Stop to check in with yourself. (See Chapter 3: Assessment.)

Assessment: *"I breathe shallow and I live shallow."*

Treatment: Take in your life more fully by taking in your breath more fully. (See Chapter 4: Hyperventilation.)

Assessment: *"I deny change going on in my life."*

Treatment: Embrace change instead of resisting or denying it. (See Chapter 5: Changing Status.)

Assessment: *"I live in the future, always thinking about the next thing I have to do."*

Treatment: Live with intention and be present to the moment. (See Chapter 6: The Treatment Plan.)

Assessment: *"I overdo my exercise, food intake, work, social life or my spending."*

Treatment: Balance the different areas in your life. (See Chapter 7: The Overdose.)

Assessment: *"I thrive on panic, chaos and crisis and often create my own emergencies."*

Treatment: Incorporate relaxation into your life. (See Chapter 8: The Adrenaline Junkie.)

Assessment: *"I always try to do everything."*

Treatment: Pace yourself more effectively. (See Chapter 9: Inserting a Pacemaker.)

Assessment: *"I do not have back-up or support systems in place."*

Treatment: Create your personal disaster plan. (See Chapter 10: The Disaster Plan.)

Assessment: *"I have trouble saying no."*

Treatment: Guard your schedule ruthlessly. (See Chapter 11: Universal Precautions.)

Assessment: *"I am feeling really burned out, resentful, and tired"*

Treatment: Take a break from your everyday life. (See Chapter 12: Take a Break.)

Assessment: *"My soul is screaming!" "I am lonely, depressed, bored."*

Treatment: Heal your emotional pain. (See Chapter 13: The Pain Scale.)

After you've selected the explanation that defines your highest priority of emergency living, reread the corresponding chapter and complete the Care Plan, even if you did it earlier. Rereading the chapter and working the Care Plan again will refresh your memory, reinforce the rescue strategies available to you, and give you the opportunity to make changes in Your Care Plan that are more appropriate this time around.

Home Care Instructions

No matter what specific area of emergency living you decide to focus on first, there are universal home care instructions to consider. These instructions are a collection of the most commonly asked questions, issues and stumbling blocks that get in our way of making lifestyle changes successfully. They are taken from my private counseling clients, my speaking audiences, and my own personal experience. These instructions will help you be successful in applying the rescue strategies to your everyday life, enabling you to change your lifestyle.

Change Your Self-Talk

The first and most critical step in overcoming your life-threatening lifestyle is giving yourself permission to make your new behaviors a priority. It's up to you to change your self-talk from "I don't have time for this" to "I am important enough to make time for this."

In shifting your self-talk, be gentle but firm with yourself. No beating yourself up or self-blaming for what you haven't done, but no excuses either. Do it *now*. You can't wait for "when things slow down," or "after the holidays," or "when you have more time." If you keep waiting, then you'll continue to wait. As Gilda Radner said, "It's always something." And it always will be.

My client Sally felt lonely and depressed, and was chronically fatigued. She said she really wanted to slow down in her life and get more sleep, get more exercise, and give herself a break, but she didn't have time. Sally never stopped. She worked late most nights at a job she hated, she volunteered for Girl Scouts, Junior League, and the soccer team, and she maintained a family household of four, meticulously, by herself. When Sally finally got ill with a debilitating autoimmune disease, she was forced to stop. She changed her self-talk to "I am important enough." She resigned from her stressful job, gave up half of her volunteer positions, and hired a housekeeper, so that she could make her own health a priority.

Focus Your Energy

Changing your lifestyle requires you to have the time and energy for your new behaviors, and this demands focus. I have talked about giving up your guilt, eliminating your drainers, and saying no—all ways of creating the space to focus on yourself. Now you have to choose what to focus your energy on. You can focus on the things you *can't* control—like the problem, the obstacles, or the final outcome. Or you can choose to focus on what you *can* control—your behaviors, your perspective, and your schedule.

You may not think something as simple as stopping for five minutes or walking for twenty requires focus, but if you don't make either one a priority and schedule time for it, chances are very good it won't happen. Introducing any new behavior into your life requires your focus. Write it down, announce it to your family, and visualize yourself doing it, whether it's going to yoga class, stopping for conscious breathing, or taking a lunch break.

Focusing your energy requires short-term planning and long-term thinking. You must focus on your schedule, your routine, or your calendar daily, keeping the "big picture" in mind. When you "don't get to something" you were planning to do, you are not focusing your energy on your plan.

Be Willing To Change

Most of us are never *really* ready to change. Changing your lifestyle requires you to change your behaviors. This may seem obvious but don't forget the definition of insanity: doing the same thing over and over again, expecting different results. How many times have you tried to slow down, quit procrastinating, or say no the exact same way, only to fail the exact same way?

It is easy to resist change because it forces us into uncomfortable and unfamiliar practices. You may never be completely ready to change, but you need to be willing to move through the discomfort, the inconvenience, and even the anxiety of change.

Change is confrontational and forces us to give something up. When we change, even if it's for the better, we suffer a loss and we must allow ourselves to grieve that loss. It is during this grieving period, or any stressful time, that we are most vulnerable, and most likely to revert to our old, comfortable behaviors.

When my clients revert to their old behaviors in the face of stress or pain, it is usually because they want to give themselves comfort. This is a universal reaction; change is hard. But in order to move beyond the pain or to deal effectively with stressful situations, you have to be willing to change and willing to be uncomfortable.

Do One Thing at a Time

My clients typically come to see me with a laundry list of issues. It isn't just one area of their life that isn't working, it is many of them. Just as I asked you to do, I ask them to identify their highest priority area of emergency living and to focus on that one first. There may be many areas in your life you want to address, too, but you have better chances for success when you focus on one behavior at a time.

Look at what happens every January when we compile our lofty list of New Year's resolutions. We all jump on the bandwagon to lose weight, eat healthy, quit smoking, clean out the garage, and take that aerobics class we've been putting off. But by mid-January the health clubs are empty, MacDonald's is back in business, the garage is still a wreck, and we're back to our same old, same old behaviors.

Don't set yourself up for failure: Be realistic, and take a hard, practical look at what behaviors you are honestly capable of changing. Choose to change, commit yourself, and then do one thing at a time.

Trust the Process

Simply stated, trusting the process means having patience and acceptance for things to take as long as they are going to take.

When you trust the process, you know you can't skip the steps. Each of us learns in different ways. Sometimes we need to learn something over and over again, or we need to learn what doesn't work before we can realize what does work. We each find our own way, in our own time.

When I counsel clients on weight management, the first question they ask is, "How long will it take me to lose the weight?" My response is always the same: "When are you going to start? When are you *really* going to start changing your behavior?" Ultimately, you're the one who determines how long it will take, when you decide to *really* start.

Trusting the process can be difficult, but when you do, it enables you to make and keep your commitments on a long-term basis, which is necessary to change your lifestyle.

Practice Daily

We become what we practice most. It takes consistent, dedicated repetition to incorporate a new behavior into your life and make it a habit. It's said that "old habits die hard." I don't think old habits die at all; they always seem to be lurking around the corner, just in case we lose our resolve.

Practice your rescue strategies every day. Practice reinforces your commitment and reminds you why you are trying to change in the first place. Practice may not make perfect, but when you don't feel like it, when it gets hard, when you lose your determination, but you practice anyway, you are changing your lifestyle.

My clients tell me when they practice their new behaviors, it's not that hard to do. It's when they "kind of" do it, or "try" to do it, that it becomes so difficult. We can either struggle to "kind of" do it, or we can build momentum, strength, and resolve with our daily practice.

My client Carla struggled for years to make lifestyle changes. She always "kind of" exercised, she "sort of" paid attention to what she was eating, she "tried not" to overcommit herself, but she never really did it, she just struggled to do it. She never made the commitment to have a daily practice of exercising, eating healthy, or saying no. When Carla finally realized how much easier it was to actually practice her behaviors daily, instead struggling to "kind of" do it, she became successful with her lifestyle changes.

Ask for Support

You can make major lifestyle changes all alone, but it is far easier when you have support from your family, friends, or even a paid professional "coach." Start with your close friends and family. Have a meeting with them and announce the new behavior you are trying to incorporate into your life, and what you need from them to help you achieve your goal. Tell them how important it is that they support you when you say "no" to their requests, when you take time for your yoga class, or when you need a break.

You always have to be accountable to yourself first, but teaming up with a counselor, coach, or a buddy for an accountability partner can contribute significantly to your success. Partners provide direction and support to help you recognize your accomplishments and keep you on track with your efforts. I have found coaching and counseling to be invaluable to me, both personally and professionally. Whether it is a structured plan with weekly meetings or acknowledgment with routine check-ins, an accountability partner can give you the support you need to be successful in making your lifestyle changes.

It's important not to disregard the many ways you are managing your life and yourself that *are* working. Sometimes we have a hard time being objective, and this is where your support systems can play a vital role in giving you a different perspective.

Define Your Stop, Start, and Continue

With every rescue strategy, there is a behavior change required. This means doing things differently. It is sometimes easier to define what we need to do if we can categorize our behaviors into what we need to *stop* doing, in order to create the space, what we need to *start* doing, to initiate a new behavior, and what we need to *continue* doing because it is already working.

○ *Stop* any behavior that gets in the way of your rescue strategy. Stop staying up so late, stop taking one more phone call in the evening, stop saying yes to unreasonable demands from your boss.

○ *Start* a new behavior that will contribute to your rescue strategy. Start scheduling time for yourself to take a walk, start practicing conscious breathing, start taking a break when you need one.

○   *Continue* any behavior that is already working for you in
     your rescue strategy. Continue to give yourself permis-
     sion, continue to make yourself a priority, keep re-
     minding yourself how you *don't* want to live
     anymore—with all of the crisis, chaos, and panic in
     your life.

Admit You Can't Start Over

When we try to change our behavior, it isn't always easy to stay
on track. When we get stressed, busy, or distracted we mind-
lessly revert to our old comfortable and familiar behaviors. I hear
so many of my clients say, " I was doing really well until my kids
got sick, or something else happened, and now I have to start all
over again."

We never start over because we are never in the same place
again. When we get off track with our new behaviors, we have
the opportunity to learn another lesson, to figure out what
doesn't work, or to be re-reminded of what gets us off track in
the first place. You pick up exactly where you left off before, not
where you first started. This is important to remember because
having to start all over again can be so overwhelming we may
decide not to do it at all.

Accept that you will get off track, because that is all part of
the process of changing our behaviors and our lifestyle. You will
have the opportunity to learn the lesson more than once, and
find out what doesn't work for you more than once. Remember
you will always be further along in your process whenever you
pick it up again; you can't start over.

Accept the Challenge

Change is hard. There is no getting around it. And changing the way we live is especially hard. The rescue strategies outlined in this book require behavior changes that are simple, but not easy.

When you accept that change is hard, you take out the element of surprise. We have all accomplished things in our lives that were hard and derived great satisfaction from our successes. Trust that the behavior changes that are hardest in the beginning will make your life all the more easy in the end.

We are never "done." We are never "there." We are never "through." This is an ongoing process of lifestyle change. Accept this challenge unconditionally by remembering why you are choosing to live a different way and overcome your life-threatening lifestyle—every day.

Identify Your Potential Obstacles

We are our own worst enemies when it comes to obstacles. We either create them ourselves or we allow someone else to create them for us. When you know what your potential obstacles are, you won't be caught off guard when they appear. You'll be prepared and able to deal with them proactively. Check the list of obstacles below. Which ones are you likely to confront as you attempt to stop living life like an emergency?

Negative Self-Talk:

- ○ I don't think I have the time.
- ○ I feel guilty about spending time on myself.
- ○ I get discouraged and give up.

Putting Yourself Last:

- ○ I allow my spouse or family to sabotage my efforts.
- ○ I don't create the space.
- ○ I feel like I have to take care of everyone else before I can focus on myself.

Going It Alone:

- ○ I think I should be able to do this alone.
- ○ I am too embarrassed to ask for help.
- ○ I don't need an accountability partner.

Unrealistic Expectations:

- ○ I try to change too many things instead of focusing on just one.
- ○ I forget how hard it is to change.
- ○ I forget how long it takes to change.

Acknowledge Your Success

You are the only one who can truly measure success for yourself. Success is the perception we have of our own progress. We must learn to appreciate all the successes we have along the way as we change our behaviors and follow through on our Care Plans.

In my one-on-one sessions with my clients, I first ask how they are doing. They immediately tell me everything they didn't do right, what didn't work, and how many mistakes they made since our last visit. I have to ask pointed questions to uncover what they have accomplished, even if it is just being more aware, so they can acknowledge their success.

I encourage my clients to follow the 80/20 rule when they define success for themselves. In the 80/20 rule, 80 percent of the time you are expected to follow your plan, focus your energy on your schedule, take your breaks, say no, or whatever other behavior change you commit to. The other 20 percent of the time you get to be human and make a mistake, slip up, forget, or revert to your old behaviors.

We don't go for perfection, because then we are sure to set ourselves up to fail. How can we realize our success? We can keep logs and document our activities. We can develop an accountability partnership and report regularly. We can do a self-assessment specific to the Care Plan we are working through.

Symptoms Requiring Your Immediate Attention

If you:

o think you are done.

o feel you no longer have a focus.

o start reverting to your old, comfortable behaviors more than 20 percent of the time.

o forget why you want to change your lifestyle and stop living life like an emergency.

o become discouraged and want to give up.

Immediately:

o Reread the corresponding chapter for your emergency living.

○ Rework your Care Plan.

○ Review your discharge instructions.

Congratulations for exploring a new way to live and following through on your discharge instructions. You undoubtedly learned some new things about yourself and were probably reminded of some things you already knew. It's not easy to take a good hard look at yourself and remain open to changing your comfortable and familiar lifestyle. I commend you for spending your time and energy on what matters most.

You now have the rescue strategies with all of the prescriptions, practical skills and instructions on how to overcome your life-threatening lifestyle. By following through on your discharge instructions, you are about to embark on a whole new way of life.

○ You will have time for the things that matter most to you.

○ You will feel better and have more energy, not only physically, but also emotionally.

○ Your relationships will be healthier and more meaningful because you have more to give.

○ You will be more productive in both your professional and personal life with a renewed sense of commitment and confidence.

○ You will be more spiritually fulfilled, because you are not only focusing on your personal belief system you are living in congruence with it.

By changing the way you live, you change the way you think, act, and react to people and situations around you. And they change too. Rejoice in your new life and the new way of living you are modeling for the rest of the world.

It is my heartfelt wish for you to continue on your path of courage, conviction, and commitment to *Stop Living Life Like an Emergency!*

> *"Whatever you can do or dream you can, begin it.*
> *Boldness has genius, magic, and power in it. Begin it now."*
> **–Goethe**

[Recommended Reading]

I could write another book about all the great books I have read, but I will list a few of my favorites that positively influenced my life. I believe that taking action with what you already know is sometimes more critical than learning more, but just in case you need more, these are my top ten recommendations.

Ban Breathnach, Sarah. *Simple Abundance* (New York: Warner Books, 1995). A daybook of comfort and joy. Through daily readings, the author shows you how your daily life can be an expression of your authentic self while taking you on a journey of your inner self. Full of creative ideas and resources, from meditations to money management, every reading will nourish a part of your soul.

Carlson, Richard. *Don't Sweat the Small Stuff...and it's all small stuff* (New York: Hyperion, 1997). Gives you simple ways to keep the little things from taking over your life. Carlson teaches you how to put things in perspective by making small daily changes such as "Do one thing at a time," or "Remember, when you die, your inbox won't be empty."

Carter-Scott, Cherie. *If Life is a Game, These Are the Rules* (New York: Broadway Books, 1998). Reviews the ten rules for being human and teaches us there are no mistakes, only lessons that are repeated. The lessons learned from each of the rules include insight on self-esteem, respect, acceptance, respect, forgiveness, ethics, compassion, humility, gratitude, and courage.

Kabat-Zinn, John. *Wherever You Go, There You Are* (New York: Hyperion, 1994). Gently walks the reader through the process of "mindfulness meditation" in everyday life. It is for both the beginner and the experienced practitioner of meditation, and includes simple and thought-provoking exercises at the end of each chapter.

Kundtz, David. *Everyday Serenity* (Berkley: Conari Press, 2000). A small book that contains a huge amount of wisdom about new ways to cope with the demands of life. Kundtz gives us brief invitations to take time for ourselves, rest, find peace, awaken, remember, and find ways to recognize what you may have forgotten. Each reading is both practical and powerful when used in your everyday life. I also recommend *Stopping: How to Be Still When You Have to Keep Going* by the same author.

Louden, Jennifer. *The Woman's Retreat Book* (San Francisco: Harper, 1997). This book was my focal point when I started facilitating my Women's Mountain Retreats. Louden not only tells women why they need to retreat, she guides them through doing it in a warm and practical way. She reminds women that nurturing themselves gives them the energy and strength they need to live full lives. I also highly recommend *The Women's Comfort Book* by the same author.

LoVerde, Mary. *Stop Screaming at the Microwave!* (New York: Fireside Books, 1998). A guide for connecting your disconnected life through the use of microactions, rethinking rituals and traditions, and instituting policies to bring tranquility into your daily life. LoVerde shows you creative ways to connect and how it improves the quality of your home life, work life, and inner life.

McGraw, Phillip C. *Life Strategies* (New York: Hyperion, 1999). A no-nonsense book to help you take control of your life by "doing what works and doing what matters." Through his Ten Laws of Life and the Seven Step Strategy, McGraw shows you how to improve virtually every aspect of your life, from work to home, spiritual to physical.

Mountain Dreamer, Oriah. *The Invitation* (San Francisco: Harper, 1999). The beginning of the poem on the front cover of this book says it all. *"It doesn't interest me what you do for a living. I want to know what you ache for, and if you dare to dream of meeting your heart's longing."* The author forces us to confront ourselves from the areas of desire and commitment to sorrow and betrayal in a most unique and unconventional way. I also recommend her sequel, *The Dance*.

St. James, Elaine. *Simplify Your Life* (New York: Hyperion, 1994). Provides 100 ways to slow down and enjoy the things that really matter, such as reduce the clutter in your life (#1), move to a smaller house (#19), or clean up your relationships (#72). St. James has a practical way of giving the permission we need to determine what is important and let the rest go. I also recommend her other books, *Simplify Your Christmas, Living the Simple Life, Simplify Your Life with Kids,* and *365 Simple Reminders.*

[Bibliography]

Brady, Maureen. *Midlife Meditations for Women*. New York: HarperCollins, 1995.

Brown, Mark. *Emergency! True Stories from the Nation's ER*. New York: St. Martin's Paperbacks, 1996.

Cameron, Julia. *The Artist's Way*. New York: G.P. Putnam's Sons, 1992.

Carlson, Richard. *Don't Sweat the Small Stuff...and it's all small stuff*. New York. Hyperion, 1997.

Domar, Alice. *Self-Nurture*. New York: Penguin Putnam, 2000.

Farhi, Donna. *The Breathing Book*. New York: Henry Holt and Company, 1996.

George, Mike. *Learn to Relax*. San Francisco: Chronicle Books, 1998.

Greene, Bob, and Oprah Winfrey. *Making the Connection: Ten Steps to a Better Body and a Better Life*. New York: Hyperion, 1996.

Hart, Archibald. *The Hidden Link Between Adrenalin and Stress. A Practical Guide to Easing Tension and Conquering Stress*. Dallas: Word Publishing, 1991.

Hendricks, Gay. *Conscious Breathing*. New York: Bantam Books, 1995.

Hudson, Janice. *Trauma Junkie: Memoirs of a Flight Nurse.*
Buffalo, NY: Firefly Books, 2001.

Iyengar, B.K.S. *Light on Pranayama: The Yogic Art of Breathing.*
New York: Crossroad Publishing Company, 1999.

Kundtz, David. *Everyday Serenity.* Berkley: Conari Press, 2000.

Louden, Jennifer. *The Woman's Retreat Book.* San Francisco:
Harper, 1997.

Loving Tubesing, Nancy, and Donald Tubesing, *Structured
Exercises in Stress Management,* Duluth, Minn. Whole
Person Press, 1994.

Mitchell, Jeff, and Grady Bray. *Emergency Services Stress:
Guidelines for Preserving the Health and Careers of
Emergency Services Personnel.* Englewood Cliffs, NJ:
Prentice-Hall, 1990.

Northrup, Christiane. *Women's Bodies, Women's Wisdom.* New
York: Bantam Books, 1994.

Weil, Andrew. *Spontaneous Healing.* New York: Ballantine
Books, 1995.

I Would Love to Hear from You!

Please feel free to share your comments, insights, and experiences about how this book helped you stop living life like an emergency and live differently. You may contact me at:

Diane Sieg

P.O. Box 2132

Estes Park, CO 80517

Voice:(970) 586-8092

Fax: (970) 577-0866

diane@dianesieg.com

www.dianesieg.com

[Index]

tardiness, 17
telephone, 119
time, taking breaks, 131–135
torso, 48
trust, in self, 164

W
warning signs, 5
work, *see* professional life

Y
"yes," postponing, 120–121